Microorganisms

Microorganisms

From Smallpox to Lyme Disease

· · ·

READINGS FROM
SCIENTIFIC AMERICAN MAGAZINE

Edited by

Thomas D. Brock
University of Wisconsin, Madison

W. H. FREEMAN AND COMPANY
New York

Some of the SCIENTIFIC AMERICAN articles in *Microorganisms: From Smallpox to Lyme Disease* are available as separate Offprints. For a complete list of articles now available as Offprints, write to Product Manager, Marketing Department, W. H. Freeman and Company, 41 Madison Avenue, New York, New York 10010.

Library of Congress Cataloging-in-Publication Data

Microorganisms: From smallpox to lyme disease: readings
    from Scientific American magazine / edited by Thomas
    D. Brock.
      p. cm.
    Includes bibliographical references.
    ISBN 0-7167-2084-1 :
    1. Medical microbiology. 2. Communicable
diseases. I. Brock, Thomas D. II. Scientific American.
    [DNLM: 1. Communicable Disease Control — collected
works. 2. Communicable Diseases — collected
works. 3. Microbiology — collected works. WC 5 M626]
QR46.M536 1990
616′.01 — dc20
DNLM/DLC
for Library of Congress   89-17205
                                  CIP

Printed in the United States of America

1 2 3 4 5 6 7 8 9 0 RRD 8 9

CONTENTS

Note on cross-references to SCIENTIFIC AMERICAN *articles:* Articles included in this book are referred to by chapter number and title; articles not included in this book but available as Offprints are referred to by title, date of publication, and Offprint number; articles not in this book and not available as Offprints are referred to by title and date of publication.

Introduction

The goal of the microbiologist is to understand how microorganisms work and through this understanding to devise ways that beneficial properties of microorganisms can be increased and harmful properties decreased. Infectious disease has always been part of human experience. Leprosy, a horribly disfiguring disease, finds common reference in the Bible, and literature and history make common reference to diseases that are still with us today. Even before microbes were known to be responsible for infectious disease, careful observation often showed that "something" was being transmitted from the sick to the well—that is, the disease was contagious. The concept of contagiousness led to the quarantining of travelers. At one time, immigrant ships entering New York harbor were held until it could be verified that passengers were free of disease. Obviously, there was something being transmitted. What was it?

Although the existence of microorganisms had been known since the 17th century, it was not until the late 19th century, through the work of Louis Pasteur and Robert Koch, that the mystery of infectious disease was swept away. Pasteur proved that the processes of putrefaction and fermentation were caused by microorganisms, and Koch proved that an infectious disease arose because of microbial growth in the human body. But Koch went further: he showed that for each specific disease there was a specific microorganism that was the cause of that disease. With improved microscopy and the development of techniques for studying microorganisms under sterile conditions, Koch described what came

to be known as "Koch's Postulates," a series of experimental procedures that could be used to prove that a particular organism caused a particular disease. Soon Koch and his students had discovered the bacteria responsible for most of the important infectious diseases of humans, including tuberculosis, cholera, diphtheria, typhoid fever and anthrax. By the end of the 19th century all of the important bacterial diseases of humans were under careful study, and the discipline of bacteriology had become an important part of the medical curriculum.

The discovery of the causes of the major infectious diseases did not lead immediately to the development of cures. Koch's discoveries did lead to several important advances: the development of methods for prevention of infectious disease through vaccination and through public health (sanitation) measures. Eventually, drugs would be discovered to treat certain infectious diseases. During World War II the first antibiotic, penicillin, was developed, and after the war there was a massive research effort by pharmaceutical companies, which led to the discovery and successful application in medicine of numerous antibiotic agents.

One measure of the success of the microbiologist and physician in conquering infectious disease is shown by the statistics in Figure I.1, which compares the present causes of death in the United States with those at the beginning of the 20th century. At the beginning of the century, the major causes of death were infectious diseases; currently, such diseases are of only minor importance in the

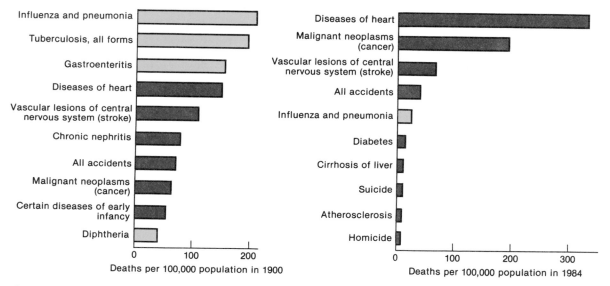

Figure I.1 DEATH RATES for the 10 leading causes of death in 1900 and 1984. Infectious diseases were the leading causes of death in 1900, whereas today they are much less important. Microbial diseases are shown in color. (From T.D. Brock, K.M. Brock and D. Ward, *Basic Microbiology with Applications*, 3rd ed., Prentice-Hall, 1986.)

United States. The exception is the tragic epidemic of acquired immunodeficiency syndrome (AIDS), which remains without cure and has a significant impact on the death rate.

This is not to say that we should no longer be concerned about infectious disease. New diseases continue to appear and old diseases continue to present new challenges. Chapter 2,"Legionellosis", and Chapter 3, "Lyme Disease," describe infectious diseases that have only been recognized in the past 20 years. Further, the United States is not typical of the world as a whole. In many parts of the world, especially in developing (Third World) countries, infectious diseases continue to remain the leading causes of death, especially of children. Several of the chapters in this book deal in some detail with diseases that are still rampant in the developing countries of Africa, Asia, Central America and South America.

Two of the heroes in this book are the U.S. Centers for Disease Control (CDC) and the World Health Organization (WHO). The CDC has been the organization on the spot during the outbreaks of the two newest diseases in the United States, legionellosis and Lyme disease. The speed with which the CDC ferreted out the causes of these two infectious diseases is truly amazing. The WHO, which is headquartered in Geneva, Switzerland, is in a sense the international counterpart of the CDC. It has led the battle to eradicate smallpox (where it was greatly abetted by the CDC), as well as other infectious diseases in the developing countries.

The chapters in this book tell some of the most interesting stories in ancient and modern medicine. They are all stories in which microorganisms, the smallest of living creatures, play major roles.

Thomas D. Brock

Microorganisms

NATURAL HISTORY OF INFECTIOUS DISEASE

. . .

Introduction to Section I

In this first section, we present the microbial connections of three infectious diseases. The first is bubonic plague, a disease no longer serious in the Western world, but one that has played a major role in human history. Called the Black Death in the Middle Ages, bubonic plague was responsible for the death of more than one-fourth of all people in Europe during the years 1346 to 1352, thus effectively changing the course of human history. Along with most of the other major bacterial diseases, plague came under medical control around the beginning of the 20th century, although it is still prevalent in certain parts of the world.

The other two diseases presented in Section I are new and effectively demonstrate that the work of the medical microbiologist is never finished. Despite vaccines, public health measures and effective antibiotics, new diseases continue to appear. The most dramatic example of this is legionellosis, also called Legionnaires' disease, which burst on the scene during a single American Legion convention in Philadelphia in the summer of 1976. Tracing the cause of this outbreak, the diligent researchers at the U.S. Centers for Disease Control discovered a completely new kind of pathogen, but one that further study showed was actually quite common. The medical detective work that led to the discovery of the cause of legionellosis makes a fascinating story.

The story of the other disease presented in Section I is less dramatic, but no less important. Lyme disease was first discovered in the area around the town of Lyme, Connecticut, in 1975. A series of fortunate circumstances led to the early discovery of the causal bacterium and the proof that it was transmitted by a tick. To date, Lyme disease appears to be restricted to only a few areas of the United States, but now that its symptoms are recognized it is likely that patients will be found in other parts of the country.

The Bubonic Plague

A bacterial disease carried by fleas that feed on rats, it has afflicted human beings for more than 1,000 years. The factors responsible for its alternate rise and fall remain a mystery.

· · ·

Colin McEvedy
February, 1988

In the year 1346 Europe, northern Africa and nearer parts of the Middle East had a total population of approximately 100 million people. In the course of the next few years a fourth of them died, victims of a new and terrifying illness that spread throughout the area, killing most of those unfortunate enough to catch it. The disease put an end to the population rise that had marked the evolution of medieval society; within four years Europe alone suffered a loss of roughly 20 million people. The disease responsible for such grim statistics was the bubonic plague, and this particular outbreak, lasting from 1346 to 1352, was known as the Great Dying or the Great Pestilence. Later it was appropriately referred to as the Black Death, a name that has come down through history.

Although the effects of the Black Death may have been particularly catastrophic, striking as it did after a long period in which the disease had been unknown in the West, this was not the first time the plague had ravaged Europe. Some 800 years earlier, during the reign of the emperor Justinian in the 6th century, there was an epidemic of similar proportions. There were also repeated, if less widespread, epidemics in the two centuries following the plague of Justinian's time, and for four centuries after the Black Death. The disease has undergone a precipitous decline since that time, but it still occurs sporadically in various parts of the world today, including the U.S.

From 70 to 80 percent of those who contracted the plague in the 14th century died from it. Indeed, the symptoms usually presented themselves with a ferocity that presaged death within five days. The name, bubonic plague, derives from one of the early signs of the disease: the appearance of large, painful swellings called buboes in the lymph nodes of the armpit, neck or groin of the victim. Three days after the appearance of the buboes people were characteristically overwhelmed by high fever, became delirious and broke out in black splotches that were the result of hemorrhaging under the skin. As the disease progressed, the buboes continued to grow larger and more painful; often they burst.

The bursting is said to have been particularly agonizing, capable of arousing even the most moribund patients to a state of frenzy. Yet physicians always regarded the bursting as a good sign, if only because it indicated that the patient was still capable of putting up a fight a week or so after the onset of the illness. Of those who were going to die, probably half were already dead by this stage.

In some cases a person's bloodstream was directly infected, which led to septic shock, massive hemorrhaging and rapid death, a form of the disease known as septicemic plague. In other cases plague was transmitted as a type of pneumonia; in pneumonic plague the victims collapsed, spit blood and were almost always dead within a few days.

Strange as it may seem, in view of the frequency of the disease and the toll it exerted on the population, no one at the time had an inkling of its fundamental nature, its ultimate cause or how it was spread. During the period of the Black Death people were inclined to attribute the disease to unfavorable astrological combinations or malignant atmospheres ("miasmas"), neither of which could be translated into a public-health program of any kind. More paranoid elaborations blamed the disease on deliberate contamination by witches, Moslems (an idea proposed by Christians), Christians (proposed by Moslems) and Jews (proposed by both groups).

It was not until 1894 that the French bacteriologist Alexandre Yersin discovered that bubonic plague is caused by a gram-negative bacterium, *Yersinia pestis*, belonging to a group of bacteria known as rod-shaped bacilli, many of which are pathogenic. Plague bacilli are found at low frequency in many wild rodent populations throughout the world and are transmitted from one rodent to another by fleas. In the case of the bubonic plague the flea often responsible for transmitting the disease is the oriental rat flea, *Xenopsylla cheopis*. When a flea bites an infected rat, it ingests the bacilli, which proceed to replicate within its digestive tract, forming a solid mass that obstructs the flea's gut; the flea is unable to ingest blood and becomes ravenously hungry. In a feeding frenzy it repeatedly bites its animal host, regurgitating plague bacilli into the host's bloodstream every time it does so. These infection sites then act as foci for the spread of bacilli. If the host animal dies, as it is likely to do, the flea moves to the next available live rodent. The disease spreads rapidly in this manner; as the number of live rats decreases, the fleas move to warm-blooded hosts on which they would not normally feed, such as human beings and their domesticated animals, and so an epidemic is launched.

Once the disease enters the human population it can sometimes spread directly from human to human through the inhalation of infected respiratory droplets. The normal mode of spread is by the bite of rat fleas, however; the disease does not persist in the absence of rodents, which are the primary hosts for both the plague bacillus and the rat flea.

The essential requirement for an epidemic (an outbreak in a human population) is a rodent epizootic (an outbreak in an animal population). This is necessary both to initiate and to sustain the disease in human beings. Of course, the two populations must be in close contact for the transmission to be successful, but it is unlikely that this was ever a significant variable in medieval times. In rural as well as urban areas humans lived surrounded by rats.

The Black Death is thought to have migrated along the Silk Road, the trans-Asian route by which Chinese silk was brought to Europe (see Figure 1.1). There are two reasons for believing this was the case. The first is that outbreaks of the plague were recorded in 1346 in Astrakhan and Saray, both caravan stations on the lower Volga River in what is now the U.S.S.R. The second is that during the years 1347 and 1348 the Arab traveler and scholar Ibn Battuta, returning along the Spice Route from a stay in India, first reported hearing news of the plague when he reached Aleppo in northern Syria, not before. That clue excludes transmission by way of the Indian Ocean and Persian Gulf ports.

Most likely the disease erupted first among marmots, large rodents native to central Asia (they are related to woodchucks but belong to a different species) whose fur was an important article of trade throughout that part of the world. According to this historical reconstruction, trappers coming across dead or dying animals collected their furs, delighted to find such an abundant supply, and sold them to dealers who in turn (without worrying about reports of illness among the fur trappers) sold them to buyers from the West. When the bales of marmot furs sent west along the Silk Road were first opened in Astrakhan and Saray, hungry fleas jumped from the fur, seeking the first available blood meal they could find. From Saray the disease is thought to have traveled down the Don River to Kaffa, a major port on the Black Sea, where a large rat population provided the perfect breeding ground for the plague bacillus. Because many of the rats in Kaffa were living on sailing vessels bound for the ports of Europe, the disease had a ready means of transport to that part of the world.

Indeed, it would be difficult to design a more

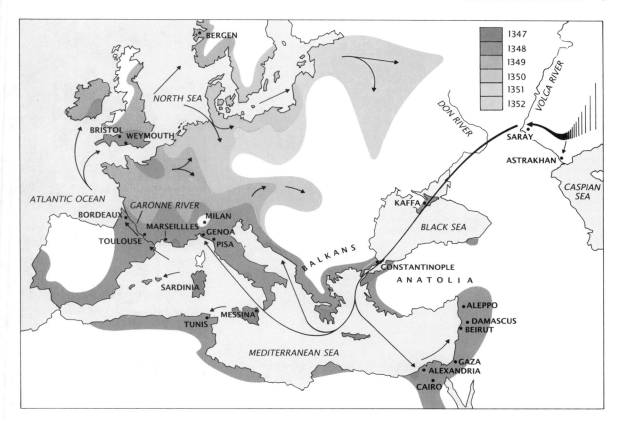

Figure 1.1 BLACK DEATH came from central Asia to Europe via the Silk Road, arriving in Kaffa in about 1347. From there it was carried by ship to the major ports of Europe and northern Africa. Most of Europe was affected before the epidemic finally subsided in 1352. Milan, the largest city to escape the plague, is believed to have done so because it is the farthest Italian city from the sea.

efficient means of disseminating the plague than a medieval ship. The holds of these ships were generally crawling with rats; when the crew slept, the rats took over, running through the rigging and dropping fleas onto the decks below. The cycle of infection, from flea to rat and rat to flea, would be maintained until the rat population was so reduced by the disease that it could no longer sustain the fleas and the plague bacteria they were carrying. Hungry fleas, seeking any host they could find, would then carry the disease into the human population. It is small wonder that by the end of 1347 plague had broken out in most ports on the route linking Kaffa to Genoa in northern Italy.

The two most important ports along this route were Pera, a suburb of Constantinople, and Messina in Sicily. Both places were stopover points for ships crossing the Mediterranean and became major foci for further dissemination of the plague. The initial impact on the population of Constantinople was graphically described by the emperor Cantacuzenus, who lost a son to the disease in 1347. He recounts how it spread throughout the Greek islands and along the coasts of Anatolia and the Balkans, killing "most of the people." In Messina the first outbreak was recorded in October of 1347, launching an epidemic that quickly spread to include the entire island.

From there in early 1348 the Black Death crossed over to Tunis on the north coast of Africa and then spread by way of Sardinia to Spain. By the time it reached Spain the Black Death had also spread to the heart of Europe, a fact that can be blamed at

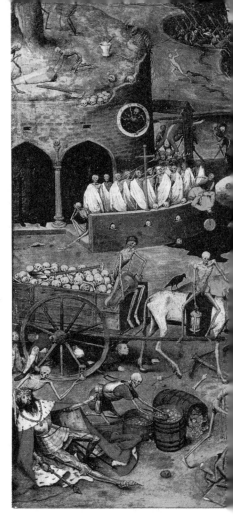

Figure 1.2 HORROR OF THE PLAGUE is captured in this 16th-century painting by Pieter Brueghel the Elder, "Triumph of Death," where death, in the form of roving skeletons, overwhelms a kingdom of the living. Neither the king with his piles of gold nor the young revelers at their table can escape the relentless army of the dead. Behind the king a corps of skeletons pushes victims into a water-filled mass grave; a barren landscape already robbed of life can be seen in the distance. Apocalyptic visions of this kind were common in the centuries when the plague ravaged Europe and the healthiest could be wiped out in a few days.

least in part on the Genoese, who are said to have heartlessly turned away ships from the east carrying their sick countrymen. Not only did such hardheartedness have little effect (the city was as badly hit as any in Europe) but also the diversion of ships to other ports, such as Marseilles and Pisa, hastened the spread of the plague throughout Europe.

By this time the epidemic was raging throughout the Mediterranean. Ships carrying silk, slaves and fur brought it to Alexandria before the end of 1347; from there it spread south to Cairo, east to Gaza, Beirut and Damascus and finally along the north coast of Africa to Morocco.

By 1348 the Black Death had jumped from the Mediterranean region to the Atlantic coast of Europe. It crossed southwestern France by way of the regional capital, Toulouse, and rapidly passed down the Garonne River to Bordeaux on the west coast. From there it is likely that one of the ships loading claret for the British market brought the Black Death to Great Britain. In 1348 it was first recorded at Weymouth on the south coast of England, and it is believed to have spread to Ireland from Bristol.

From England the plague crossed the North Sea to envelop Scandinavia in its deadly grasp. According to one story, the invasion of Scandinavia can be blamed on a ship that left London in May, 1349, bound for Bergen with a full crew and a cargo of wool. The ship is reported to have been seen some days later, drifting off the coast of Norway. Local people who rowed out to investigate found the crew dead and returned to shore, carrying the wool and

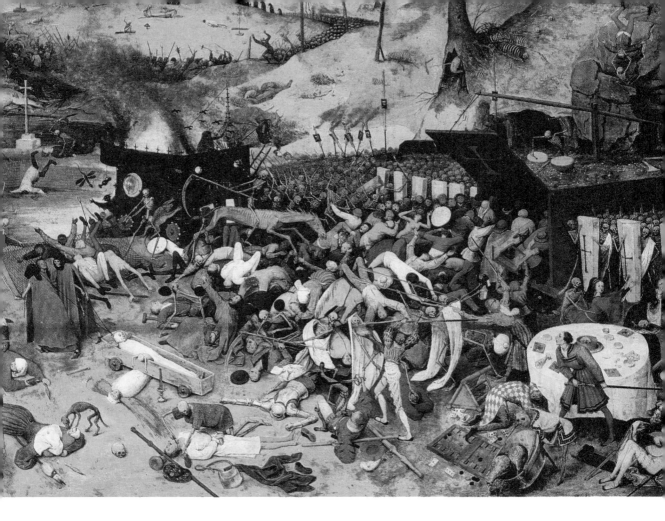

—unwittingly—the plague with them. That started a chain reaction as village after village along the Norwegian coast succumbed to the disease.

The following year the Black Death ravaged the populations of Denmark and Germany before entering Poland in 1351 and Russia in 1352. This in effect completed the circle; not only had the disease returned to within a few hundred miles of its entry into Europe on the Volga steppe but also after four long and devastating years mortality rates in western Europe had finally returned to normal.

The society that emerged from the period of the Black Death became quite prosperous; the survivors had inherited the fortunes of their deceased relatives and many were able to move into positions of prominence once closed to them. Their good fortune did not necessarily last for long, however. In 1356 a second outbreak of the plague appeared in Germany and spread rapidly throughout Europe. It exacted a particularly heavy toll among the children born since the end of the Black Death.

Thereafter the plague returned to Europe with mournful regularity; indeed, the continent never seemed free of it for more than a few years at a time. Although the later epidemics never matched the Black Death in terms of overall mortality, they nonetheless continued to have a negative impact on population growth in Europe through the end of the 14th century. Figure 1.2 illustrates an artist's conception of the ravages of plague in the 16th century.

At this point an equilibrium was reached between

plague and people, and in the 15th century the population began to recover. In particularly hard-hit regions it took more than a century for numbers to return to their original levels, but by the end of the 16th century populations all over were higher than they had been prior to the onset of the Black Death.

Strangely, when the plague did reappear (which it continued to do, albeit less frequently), it often did so with a ferocity equal to any recorded in previous outbreaks. In the last epidemic in France, from 1720 to 1722, half of the population of the city of Marseilles died, together with 60 percent of the population in neighboring Toulon, 44 percent at Arles and 30 percent at Aix and Avignon (see Figure 1.3). Yet the epidemic did not spread beyond Provence, and the total number of deaths was less than 100,000.

By the 16th century it was widely believed the plague spread as a result of contagion: a toxic factor that could be transferred from the sick to the healthy. Human-to-human transmission was

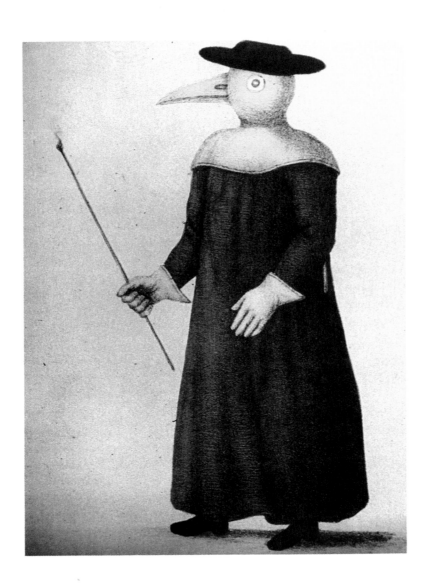

Figure 1.3 PHYSICIAN'S GARB that was worn during a plague outbreak in Marseilles in 1720. The birdlike costume, made of leather, covered its wearer from head to toe and was believed to provide protection from contagion. The large beak contained sweet-smelling herbs to filter airborne contagion; the wand contained incense that was thought to ward off impurities. Even the eyeholes, which held crystalline lenses, were protective.

thought to take place either directly through physical contact with a sick person or indirectly by the clothes or bed sheets. In response, many towns and villages instituted quarantine regulations. The authorities in England, for example, recommended that plague victims be locked up in their homes or transferred to special "pest houses." An extreme example of adherence to public policy is the famous case of William Mompesson, rector in the small village of Eyam in Derbyshire, who persuaded the entire community to enter into quarantine when the plague erupted there in 1666. One by one the parishioners who remained faithful to their contaminated hearths fell victim to the disease. A mortality rate of 72 percent indicates that the community probably had a morbidity (infection) rate of 100 percent, an extraordinary price to pay for a misconceived theory.

Locking people in their homes is, of course, one of the worst possible ways to fight the plague. The plague is a disease of "locality," most likely to manifest itself when rats, fleas and people are kept in close contact with one another (see Figure 1.4). To confine people is to maximize their chance of being bitten by a plague-carrying flea or infected through close contact with another human being.

Officials recognized that quarantines were dangerous to healthy individuals confined with sick

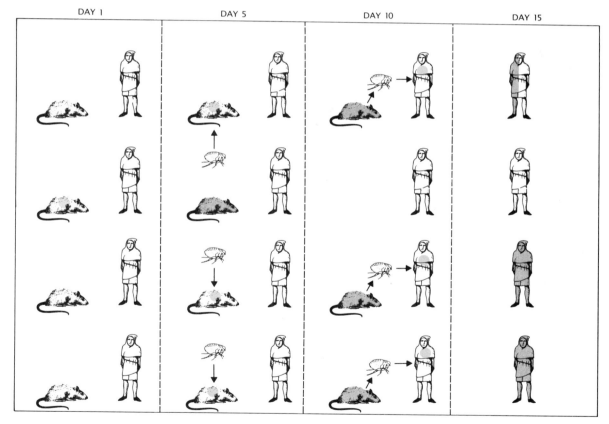

Figure 1.4 PROGRESSION OF THE PLAGUE through a medieval household could be very rapid once the black rats that lived there became infected. An infected rat, marked with a colored dot on day 1, is shown to die from the disease by day 5 and its fleas leave, carrying the plague with them to other rats in the house. By day 10 these rats have also died and the fleas turn to human beings, infecting almost 75 percent of them. By day 15 approximately half of the humans in the house will have died from the plague; a fourth of them will have recovered from it and a fourth will have escaped it.

relatives, but they imposed them nonetheless in the belief that some lives must be sacrificed in order to stop further spread of the disease. Because it is rats that carry the plague (and the rats were free to travel), the entire quarantine effort was a waste of time—and lives.

Attempts were also made to quarantine passengers and goods arriving in boats from overseas. When sickness suggestive of the plague was observed among crew members or passengers, the ships were diverted to lazarettos (quarantine stations) until the authorities deemed it safe to release them. At Marseilles in May of 1720, for example, the sailing ship *Grand Saint Antoine* was placed in quarantine for three weeks because eight of its crew had died in the course of the voyage from the Near East. In spite of these efforts to limit the spread of the plague, the disease broke out in Marseilles—first among the dockworkers who unloaded the ship's cargo when it was released from quarantine and then in the population at large.

There is little evidence that quarantines of this type were ever very effective. Venice was one of the first seaports to introduce quarantine regulations, early in the 15th century, enforcing them by imposing the death penalty on anyone who broke the rules. Yet Venice suffered from the plague as much as any city in Italy, presumably because it was impossible to prevent rats aboard quarantined ships from jumping ashore, carrying the plague with them.

Finally, after innumerable cycles of onslaught and retreat, the plague disappeared from Europe. London's last experience with the disease, the Great Plague, began in 1665 and ended in spectacular fashion with the Great Fire of 1666. At that time it was natural of Londoners to believe they owed their deliverance to the purifying conflagration. Later it was suggested Londoners owed their resistance to the plague to the reconstruction that followed the fire and the fact that the rebuilt city boasted brick houses and wide, rubbish-free streets in place of the higgledy-piggledy structures and malodorous alleys of medieval times.

This explanation is attractive but does not hold up under scrutiny. One reason is that the fire destroyed only the central part of London, the area least affected by any of the outbreaks of plague earlier in the century, leaving untouched the overcrowded suburbs that had provided the disease with its main lodging in previous times. A second reason is that

other cities in Europe, such as Paris and Amsterdam, became plague-free during the same period—a phenomenon that could not be linked to the Great Fire of London.

A somewhat more convincing (but still flawed) theory suggests that the disappearance of the plague coincided with a slow rise in prevailing standards of health and hygiene. Although hygiene cannot be eliminated as a factor, it does not explain why subsequent outbreaks followed the standard course, complete with high rates of mortality, but were farther and farther away from the center of Europe each time they appeared. It was almost as if Europe were developing some form of resistance to the plague that kept the infection from propagating in the usual way. In the north the path of retreat was to the east; in the Mediterranean it was to the south. The later the epidemic, the less it seemed to be capable of spreading. This, moreover, was at a time when, according to every available index, traffic by land and by sea was increasing.

When the role of rats was finally established late in the 19th century, it was suggested that the subsidence of the plague could be explained by changes in the population dynamics of the black rat, *Rattus rattus*. During the 18th century it had been observed that the black rat, the historic carrier, had been largely displaced by a new species, the brown rat (*Rattus norvegicus*), which would have been a much poorer vector of the plague: the brown rat is as susceptible to the plague bacillus as the black rat but does not normally live in close proximity to humans. Brown rats typically live in dark cellars or sewers, whereas black rats overrun the upper rooms and rafters of a house. Because the oriental rat flea has a maximum jump of 90 millimeters (a little more than 3.5 inches), the difference in preferred habitats may have been enough to isolate humans from plague-infested fleas.

The brown-rat theory seems plausible but does not fit the geography: the brown rat spread across Europe in the 18th century from east to west, whereas the plague retreated from west to east. The brown rat was in Moscow long before the city experienced a particularly severe epidemic of the plague in the 1770's; it did not reach England until 1727, more than 60 years after that country's last bout of the plague.

The late Andrew B. Appleby of San Diego State University suggested an alternative theory, namely that a certain percentage of black rats became resistant to the plague over the course of the 17th century and that the resistant animals would have increased in number, spreading across Europe during the next 100 years. Although these rats might still be infected by the plague bacillus, they would not die from it and therefore could support a large population of fleas, rendering it unnecessary for the fleas to seek other hosts. This theory, however, does not conform to what is known about resistance to plague in animal populations. As Paul Slack of the University of Oxford has pointed out, rat populations often develop resistance when exposed to a pathogenic bacterium or virus, but such resistance is short-lived and is therefore unlikely to have been responsible for broad-based immunity to the plague.

A more plausible theory suggests that a new species of plague bacillus, *Yersinia pestis*, may have evolved that was less virulent than the previous strain. Being less virulent, it might have acted as a vaccine, conferring on infected animals and humans a relative immunity to more virulent strains of the bacterium.

The bacteriological theory is acceptable on several grounds. First, it conforms to the dictum, proposed by the American pathologist Theobold Smith, that "pathological manifestations are only incidents in a developing parasitism," so that in the long run milder forms of disease tend to displace more virulent ones. Second, it explains why the decline of the plague is associated with a failure to spread beyond local outbreaks: a disease cannot travel far when the number of people susceptible to it is low. Third, it is supported by the existence of a close relative of the plague bacillus, *Yersinia pseudotuberculosis*, which does not induce visible illness in rats but does confer on them a high degree of immunity to the plague.

Did *Y. pseudotuberculosis*, or a relative with similar properties, gradually spread through the rodent population of early modern Europe, making it impossible for *Y. pestis* to gain a foothold there? Although no direct evidence exists to support that hypothesis, it seems more reasonable than any other.

The discovery and widespread use of antibiotics has conferred on human beings a different form of protection from the plague. Although the disease still occurs with regularity throughout parts of Africa, South America and the southwestern U.S. (in 1986, 10 cases were reported in the U.S.), it is never again likely to reach epidemic levels now that we know how it spreads, what public-health mea-

sures are appropriate and how to treat plague cases as they occur. Nevertheless, many questions about the plague are as yet unanswered. For example, the mode of transmission in rural areas, where rat populations are discontinuous, is entirely unclear. And what explains the distribution of the plague throughout the world today? Why are only certain rodent populations reservoirs of the disease whereas others are entirely free of it?

POSTSCRIPT

Although the word "plague" is often used generally to refer to any human affliction, bubonic plague is a specific disease caused by a specific bacterium named *Yersinia pestis*. One of the most feared diseases, the name Black Death is linked to a major epidemic of bubonic plague that decimated the civilized world in the years between 1346 and 1352. Although human society had certainly been ravaged by infectious disease earlier, the Black Death was the first widespread epidemic for which sufficient records exist so that its extent and course can be tracked. Coming at a time when human society was wrapped up in the superstitions of the Middle Ages, the Black Death was linked with all manner of fanciful causes, or with minority groups. For instance, a woodcut of the times shows Jews being rounded up and burned because it was thought that they were guilty of spreading the plague.

From an ecological viewpoint, plague is one of the most interesting infectious diseases because normally it is not a disease of humans at all. The Black Death and the later episodes of bubonic plague were the unfortunate result of accidental association of humans with rats and with the fleas that accompany rats. Although the plague was a mild disease of rats, when it spread to humans in the Middle Ages it assumed a new and particularly malevolent form.

Why was it the "black" death? We now know that the bacterium that causes plague produces a toxin that causes the destruction of blood vessels. As the blood oozes from the capillaries into the surrounding tissues, hemorrhage and fluid accumulation occur, resulting in oedomatous swellings. Gangrene develops, especially in the extremities, with vicious-looking black lesions on the hands and legs. Although the worldwide epidemics of the plague have long since ceased, the disease is still found in numerous countries in Africa, Asia, North America and South America. In the first 20 years of the 20th century, over 12 million people died of the plague in India alone. There are still occasional cases in the United States, generally concentrated in the Southwest and Rocky Mountain regions, associated not with rats but with wild rodents.

Among the more interesting ideas is the suggestion that the bacterium which causes plague, *Yersinia pestis*, may have changed its virulence in the centuries since the great scourge of the Black Death. It is often thought that the most successful disease-causing microorganisms are those that live in "harmony" with their hosts. Of what advantage is it to the pathogen to kill its host? Evolutionary success for a pathogen requires that it multiply and produce numerous offspring and since only when it is in a living host is the pathogen able to grow and reproduce, common sense will dictate that killing the "goose that laid the golden egg" is not the proper thing to do. Many ecologists believe that in the early stages of the development of a disease, the pathogen may be unusually virulent, but gradually reduces its virulence as it becomes more "adapted" to its host. This type of adaptation may have happened with *Yersinia pestis*, and if so, this would explain why violent epidemics, such as that of the Black Death, no longer occur.

As with other bacterial diseases, the advent of antibiotics has changed the whole medical picture. Diagnosed in time, therapy of plague is almost universally successful. The most effective antibiotic is streptomycin, but tetracycline, kanamycin and sulfadiazine can also be used. Although vaccines (see Section II) for plague are available, they are only used with people in high-risk areas, such as laboratory personnel working with virulent cultures.

Fortunately, plague is primarily of historical interest today, although it was at one time considered as a biological warfare agent (see Chapter 12), but it teaches us much about epidemics (see Chapter 11) —how they spread and how they are controlled.

Legionellosis

The mysterious 1976 Legionnaires' disease epidemic has been traced to a previously unknown bacterium. Legionellosis, the infection the bacterium gives rise to, has turned out to be not very rare after all.

. . .

David W. Fraser and Joseph E. McDade
October, 1979

The 58th annual convention of the American Legion's Pennsylvania Department was held at the Bellevue-Stratford Hotel in Philadelphia from July 21 through 24, 1976. In most respects it was a typical Legion convention, with some 4,400 delegates, members of their families and other conventioneers on hand for a parade, meetings and the variety of social activities, formal and informal, that are customary on such occasions. What no one realized was that this convention was destined to be recorded in the annals of medicine. Between July 22 and August 3, 149 of the conventioneers developed what appeared to be the same puzzling illness, characterized by fever, coughing and pneumonia. This, however, was an unusual, explosive outbreak of pneumonia, with no apparent cause. Because most of the conventioneers had returned to their homes before becoming ill it was not until August 2 that reports to the Pennsylvania Department of Health made it clear that an epidemic had developed among those who had attended the convention.

That day marked the start of one of the largest and most complex investigations of an epidemic ever undertaken. Legionnaires' disease, as the illness was quickly named by the press, was to prove a formidable challenge to epidemiologists and laboratory investigators alike. Only after many months was the causative agent discovered, and more months were to pass before the agent was characterized as a previously unknown bacterium. Meanwhile Legionnaires' disease had been shown to be not a rare illness but a relatively common one, responsible for other outbreaks and for sporadic individual cases in many parts of the world both before the Philadelphia epidemic and after it.

EPIDEMIOLOGY

The initial step in the investigation of any epidemic is to determine the characteristics of the illness, who has become ill and just where and when. The next step is to find out what was unique about the people who became ill: where they were and what they did that was different from other people in the same general group who stayed well. Knowing such things may indicate how the disease agent was spread and thereby suggest the identity of the agent and where it came from. In order to gather such information as quickly as possible from conventioneers dispersed throughout the state 23 epidemic intelligence officers from the Centers for Disease

Control (CDC) of the U.S. Public Health Service collaborated with scores of public-health workers from the Pennsylvania and Philadelphia health departments.

We quickly learned that the illness was not confined to Legionnaires. An additional 72 cases were discovered among people who had not been directly associated with the convention. They had one thing in common with the sick conventioneers: for one reason or another they had been in or near the Bellevue-Stratford Hotel. All together 221 people had become ill; 34 of them died of pneumonia or its complications.

Older conventioneers had been affected at a higher rate than younger ones, men at three times the rate for women. Legionnaires who had stayed overnight at the Bellevue-Stratford showed a higher illness rate than those who stayed elsewhere, and among the latter those who became ill had spent more time at that hotel than those who remained well (see Figure 2.1). The only family contacts who became ill had themselves been in Philadelphia for the convention, indicating that the disease had not been spread from person to person. The distribution of cases suggested that a common source was responsible for the outbreak (see Figure 2.2), but the obvious possibility that the disease might have been spread by food or drink was ruled out. Conventioneers who became ill were shown to be no more likely than those who remained well to have eaten at particular restaurants, to have attended particular functions where food and drink were served or to have drunk water or used ice in the hotels.

Certain observations suggested that the disease might have been spread through the air. Legionnaires who became ill had spent on the average about 60 percent more time in the lobby of the Bellevue-Stratford than those who remained well; the sick Legionnaires had also spent more time on the sidewalk in front of the hotel than their unaffected fellow conventioneers. If the disease agent had contaminated the air in the lobby and passed through the front door to the sidewalk, it could have affected Legionnaires and other hotel visitors in just that pattern. It appeared, therefore, that the most likely mode of transmission was airborne. What agent had caused the disease, however, remained undetermined for some time.

FINDING THE AGENT

The clinical symptoms could have been caused by a wide variety of agents, including heavy metals, toxic organic substances and infectious organisms.

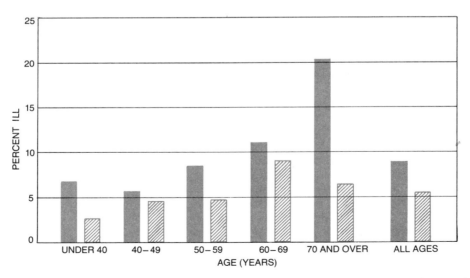

Figure 2.1 ATTACK RATE in the 1976 Legionnaires' disease epidemic varied among delegates to the Philadelphia convention with age and hotel of residence. The incidence was higher for older Legionnaires than it was for younger ones and also higher for delegates who stayed at the Bellevue-Stratford Hotel (*solid color bars*) than it was for those who stayed at other hotels (*hatched bars*).

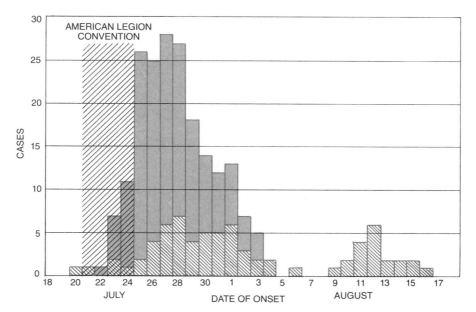

Figure 2.2 DISTRIBUTION OF CASES in the Philadelphia epidemic was typical of an outbreak arising from a common source: the number of cases among conventioneers (*color*) and among other people (*color hatching*) rose rapidly from July 22 through July 25 and later declined more slowly. The relation between the dates of the convention and the onset of illness among Legionnaires indicated that the incubation period of Legionnaires' disease ranged from two to 10 days.

During the first weeks of the investigation specimens obtained from patients and tissues taken at autopsy were subjected to intensive testing. Comparison of specimens from cases and controls failed to reveal the consistent presence in patients of unusual levels of metallic or toxic organic substances that might be related to the epidemic; no known microbial agents were found that could explain the outbreak. The testing continued, however, with attention directed to the possibility that some unknown organism had been responsible but had somehow escaped detection. That supposition turned out to be correct.

In January, 1977, in collaboration with Charles C. Shepard and others at the CDC, we isolated from the tissues of Legionnaires who had died of the disease a previously unrecognized pathogenic bacterium and then identified it as the causative agent. How the bacterium had escaped earlier detection became clear only after it had been isolated and characterized.

The agent was discovered not during an attempt to isolate a bacterium but rather by a procedure designed to isolate a rickettsia, a very small bacteriumlike organism. Rickettsias are special in that they do not grow on synthetic culture mediums as most bacteria do but grow only in a living host such as the anthropods many of them parasitize, experimental animals such as guinea pigs and embryonated eggs. One rickettsia species, *Coxiella burnetii*, causes a type of pneumonia called Q fever. Attempting to isolate *C. burnetii*, we inoculated guinea pigs with tissue specimens obtained from patients at autopsy. The guinea pigs developed fever; after several days they were sacrificed, and microscopic examination of stained tissue samples yielded a first result. A spleen specimen stained by the Giménez technique contained some small rod-shaped organisms (see Figure 2.3).

That observation in itself did not mean very much. The presence of a few organisms in the guinea pig spleen was far from establishing that they had caused the patient's death, but it did provide a promising lead. In order to enhance the growth of the organisms and any other present in the animals' tissues, suspensions of guinea pig

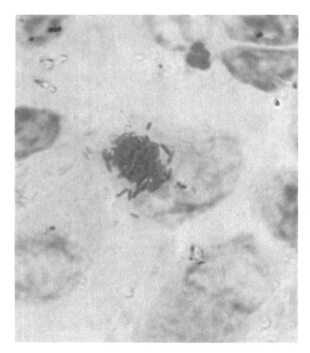 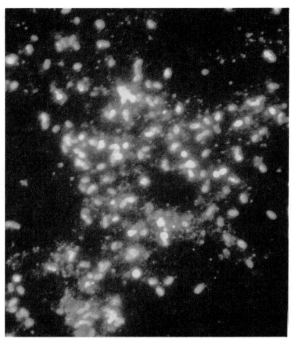

Figure 2.3 AGENT OF LEGIONNAIRES' DISEASE was first observed in a smear of the spleen of a guinea pig inoculated with lung tissue from a patient who died of the disease. The micrograph (*left*) reveals rod-shaped organisms stained red, which were shown to be bacteria when they were grown on a modified bacteriologic me- dium and shown to have caused Legionnaires' disease by indirect fluorescent-antibody tests (*see Figure 2.5*). In a similar test, suspensions of diseased lung tissue are stained with a fluorescein-linked rabbit antibody to the Legionnaires' disease agent. The antibody becomes fixed to the bacterium and the bacteria glow yellow green (*right*).

spleen were inoculated into the yolk sac of embryonated hen eggs. The embryos died several days later. The yolk-sac membranes were harvested and smears of the membranes were stained by the Giménez method. An apparently pure culture of rod-shaped organisms (bacilli) was visible in the yolk-sac smears (see Figure 2.4). We could not tell whether they were large rickettsias or small bacteria, but we immediately proceeded to find out if they were the cause of Legionnaires' disease.

ESTABLISHING CAUSE

We did that by testing the serums of the Legionnaires' disease patients for antibodies to the newly isolated organism. When a patient's serum is found to contain antibodies specific for the antigen molecules on a given organism, it is said to be "seroposi-

tive"; one can assume then that the patient has been exposed to that particular organism (or possibly one with similar antigens) at some time. If the patient's antibody level is found to have risen in the course of convalescence from a given illness, "seroconversion" has been demonstrated and it is very likely that the illness was caused by the particular organism.

When we tested serums from the Legionnaires' disease patients for antibodies to the newly isolated organism by indirect fluorescent-antibody tests (see Figure 2.5), more than 90 percent of the serum specimens taken during convalescence turned out to be seropositive. In more than 50 percent of the cases — most of those for which suitably timed serum specimens were available — we were able to demonstrate seroconversion, indicating that the patients had recently been infected by this particular bacillus.

Although the results of the indirect fluorescent-antibody tests showed that we had isolated the causative agent of Legionnaires' disease, for several weeks we did not know whether the organism was a rickettsia or a bacterium. Morphologically it appeared to be a bacterium, but it had been isolated by techniques more appropriate to rickettsias, and it failed to grow on a variety of culture mediums on which bacteria normally thrive. Then, finally, Robert E. Weaver of the CDC found a bacteriologic medium on which the bacillus would grow. It was similar to the one on which gonococci are isolated, and it was prepared by adding 1 percent hemoglobin and 1 percent of a commercial supplement (IsoVitaleX) to a standard medium (Mueller-Hinton agar). When Weaver inoculated this medium with a heavy suspension of infected yolk-sac material, distinct bacterial colonies were observed growing on the culture plates after several days of incubation. The newly isolated bacillus was thereby shown to be not a rickettsia but rather a bacterium.

It was an exceedingly fastidious bacterium, with very specific growth requirements. James C. Feeley and his associates at the CDC defined the requirements. Among other things, the bacterium will not grow unless the medium contains a high enough concentration of the amino acid cysteine (of which IsoVitaleX has a large amount) and of iron (which was supplied by the hemoglobin). Such specific nutritional constraints are unusual. Many bacteria require supplementary cysteine or iron for growth, but the double requirement is rare.

Another unusual characteristic of the Legionnaires' disease bacterium is that in pathologic specimens (lung tissue from a patient, for example) it cannot consistently be stained by techniques that normally are effective for bacteria. Even after it was established (by our successful isolation of the organism from lung tissue) that the bacteria were present in diseased lungs, the organisms could still not be seen in lung sections stained by the usual methods. Francis W. Chandler and his colleagues at the CDC thereupon tried a number of less conventional methods. Eventually they found that the bacterium could be stained dependably by a modification of the Dieterle silver-impregnation technique, a procedure developed more than 50 years ago for staining the spirochete of syphilis. The many unusual properties of the Legionnaires' disease bacterium suggested it was an unknown species, but more detailed characterization of the organism was necessary before that could be established.

EARLIER OUTBREAKS

Meanwhile another line of research being pursued in the course of the intensive CDC investigation was producing evidence that the bacterium was new only in the sense that it was unfamiliar to laboratory workers. An important question presented by the original discovery of the agent was whether or not the unfamiliar bacillus had been responsible for earlier outbreaks of respiratory disease for which no cause had ever been discovered. Perhaps the most notorious of those outbreaks was the outbreak of "Pontiac fever" in 1968. Beginning on July 2 of that year 95 of the 100 people who worked in a single building of the Oakland County Health Department in Pontiac, Mich., developed high fever, headache and muscle aches; other common symptoms were diarrhea, vomiting and chest pain, but there was no pneumonia. The illness lasted for only three or four days and all patients recovered. A team of CDC epidemiologists headed by Thomas H. Glick and Michael B. Gregg went to investigate the outbreak, and several of them became ill a day or two after entering the building. Guinea pigs exposed to the air in the building by Arnold F. Kaufmann developed pneumonia, whereas control animals placed in adjacent buildings remained healthy.

It was noted that of all the people who entered the building, the only ones spared were those who were there only when the air-conditioning system was turned off. Investigation of the air-conditioning system disclosed a defect. Mist generated by the evaporative condenser was not being exhausted properly; holes in an exhaust vent and a fresh-air vent had allowed the mist to condense and accumulate in a puddle in the fresh-air duct. Guinea pigs exposed to an aerosol of water from the puddle developed pneumonia. The conclusion reached at the time was that the agent of Pontiac fever was in the evaporative-condenser water and had been spread by the air-conditioning system. No pathogenic organisms could be isolated, however, and the cause of the illness remained undetermined.

Serum specimens collected from Pontiac fever patients had been preserved at the CDC. In 1977, nine years later, they were tested for antibodies to the newly isolated Legionnaires' disease bacillus. Serum specimens from 31 of 37 cases showed servoconversion to the organism during convalescence, indicating that Pontiac fever had been caused by the same agent that caused Legionnaires' disease.

Another earlier outbreak traced to the same

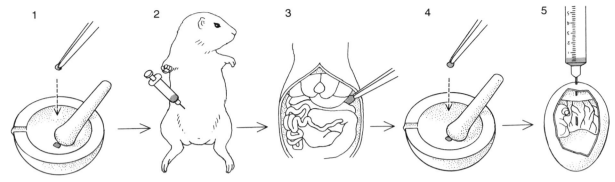

Figure 2.4 TO ISOLATE THE BACTERIUM a bit of lung tissue from a patient was ground up (1) and inoculated into the abdominal cavity of guinea pigs (2). At autopsy (3) a bit of spleen tissue was made into a suspension (4) that was inoculated into the yolk sacs of embryonated eggs (5) to enhance the growth of any organism present. The embryos died in four or five days. The yolk-sac membrane was removed (6), smeared on a microscope slide (7) and stained (8). Rod-shaped organisms were visible under the microscope (9). A yolk-sac membrane was made into a suspension (10), which was streaked on various bacteriologic mediums (11). Bacterial colonies eventually grew on an enriched Mueller-Hinton agar (12).

organism dated back to July and August of 1965, when 81 patients at St. Elizabeth's Hospital, a chronic-care facility in Washington, D.C., developed pneumonia and 14 died. The cause could not be determined. In 1977 paired acute-phase and convalescent-phase serum specimens from 23 patients were tested against the Legionnaires' disease agent. For 17 patients there was a substantial rise in antibodies to the bacterium. Similar results associated the bacterium with several other earlier outbreaks, including one that had affected Scottish vacationers at a Spanish resort in 1973.

Publication of a report on the characteristics of the Legionnaires' disease bacterium also led to the production of direct evidence of earlier infection by the same agent. F. Marilyn Bozeman of the U.S. Food and Drug Administration noticed that the bacterium was similar in some respects to four hitherto unclassified rickettsialike agents she had described years before. Like the newly isolated bacterium, each of them had been isolated in embryonated eggs from guinea pigs inoculated with clinical or autopsy specimens and each could be stained by the Giménez method. From the time of Bozeman's investigations the unidentified agents had been stored in a deep freeze. In 1978 various tests revealed that three of the four rickettsialike agents were not related to the Legionnaires' disease agent but that the fourth was virtually identical with it. The identical bacterium had been isolated in 1947 from a guinea pig inoculated with blood from a patient who had a febrile respiratory illness.

CHARACTERIZING THE BACTERIUM

Meanwhile the effort to learn more about the Legionnaires' disease bacterium continued. Before a bacterium is designated as a new species one must show convincingly that it is significantly different from all previously described species. A team of CDC microbiologists examined the newly isolated bacterium's morphology, physiology and staining characteristics, its susceptibility to various antibiotics, its antigens and its fatty-acid composition. Under the electron microscope the bacterium looked structurally similar to many other bacteria (see Figure 2.6), but study of other characteristics soon showed it was a completely new organism. These characteristics were then compared with those of known bacteria. The Legionnaires' disease agent turned out to have quite a few properties in common with other bacteria, but the overall pattern of its properties was quite different from that of any known species.

Convincing evidence that the organism was a new species came when Donald J. Brenner, Arnold G. Steigerwalt and their CDC colleagues compared the genetic material of the Philadelphia bacterium with that of other bacteria by means of the elegant DNA-hybridization technique (see Figure 2.7). The chromosome of the Legionnaires' disease bacte-

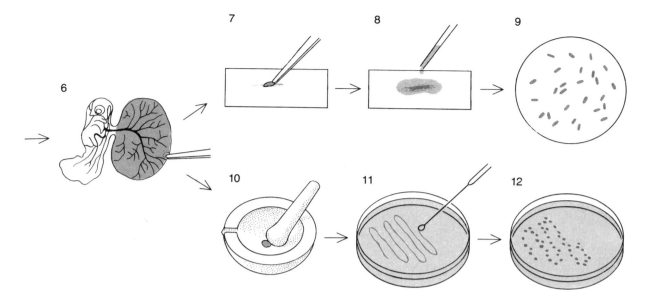

rium, like that of other bacteria, is a double-strand DNA molecule composed of two single strands linked by base pairing between complementary nucleotides. Under the appropriate experimental conditions single strands of DNA from related species can combine to form hybrid double-strand molecules; the degree of hybridization depends on the closeness of the relation.

Attempts to hybridize single strands of DNA from the Legionnaires' disease bacterium with single strands from many other bacteria failed to identify any species that were related to the newly isolated organism. Although additional comparisons are still being made, the available evidence seems to justify the designation of the bacterium as a new genus and species. It has provisionally been named *Legionella pneumophila*.

In retrospect it is easy to understand how *L. pneumophila* had remained undetected even though it has been causing illness for decades. First of all, the disease it causes is clinically similar to several types of nonbacterial ("atypical") pneumonia, and in searching for the agents of such diseases investigators commonly add antibiotics to the specimens to reduce contamination by bacteria. This makes it easier to isolate a virus or rickettsia, if either is the culprit, but it usually precludes the recovery of bacteria such as *L. pneumophila*. The bacterium was finally isolated in the course of a rickettsial isolation procedure in which no antibiotics were included.

Second, the peculiar growth requirements of the bacterium had militated against its earlier identification. The mediums on which the usual pneumonia-causing bacteria or fungi are ordinarily isolated do not contain the optimal concentrations of cysteine and iron. Finally, the inability to consistently visualize the bacterium in tissue stained by the usual methods had surely been a major obstacle for workers investigating earlier cases of atypical pneumonia that were caused by *L. pneumophila*.

CLINICAL COURSE AND THERAPY

Legionellosis, as illness caused by *L. pneumophila* is now designated, has so far been seen in two basic forms: Legionnaires' disease and Pontiac fever (see Figure 2.8). The clear distinguishing features are the incubation period, the attack rate and the presence of pneumonia.

Legionnaires' disease typically begins from two to 10 days after exposure. A general feeling of malaise is accompanied by muscle aches and a slight headache. The fever rises rapidly and is usually accompanied by coughing, chest and abdominal pain, diarrhea and shortness of breath. When patients are first seen by a physician, most of them have a temperature of from 102 to 105 degrees Fahrenheit and pulmonary rales (abnormal breathing sounds heard with a stethoscope, suggesting pulmonary infection). Some patients appear confused or stuporous,

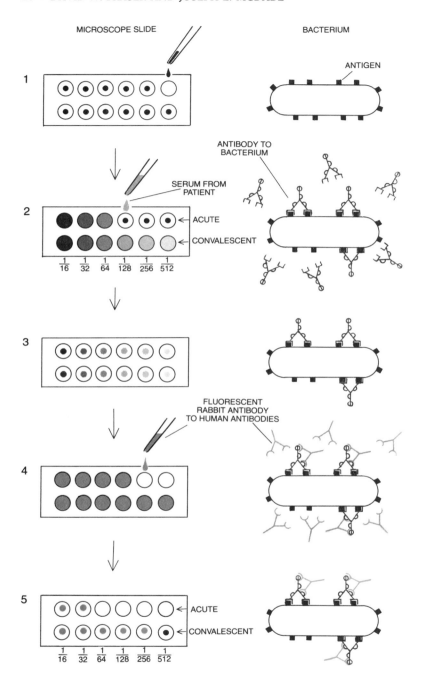

Figure 2.5 INDIRECT FLUORES-
CENT-ANTIBODY TEST at the
experimental level (*left*) and at the
level of the organism (*right*). A
drop of infected yolk-sac membrane was placed in each of 12
wells on a slide (*1*) and dilutions
of serum taken from a patient
during the acute and convalescent
phases were placed in each set of
six wells (*2*); any antibody (*gray
Y-shaped structures*) to the bacterium in the serum became fixed to
antigens on the outer membrane.
The slides were washed (*3*), and a
fluorescein-labeled rabbit antibody (*color*) to human antibodies
was added (*4*); the rabbit antibody
attached to whatever patient antibodies had remained fixed to the
bacterium. Bacteria with antibodies attached emitted a yellow-
green glow under the microscope
(*5*).

suggesting that the central nervous system may be
affected. Tests usually show a moderately elevated
white-blood-cell count, an increased number of immature cells, a high red-cell sedimentation rate,
protein and red cells in the urine and evidence of

some abnormalities of liver and kidney function. In
90 percent of the patients chest radiographs show
pneumonia.

Patients with Legionnaires' disease usually require hospitalization, and for several days after ad-

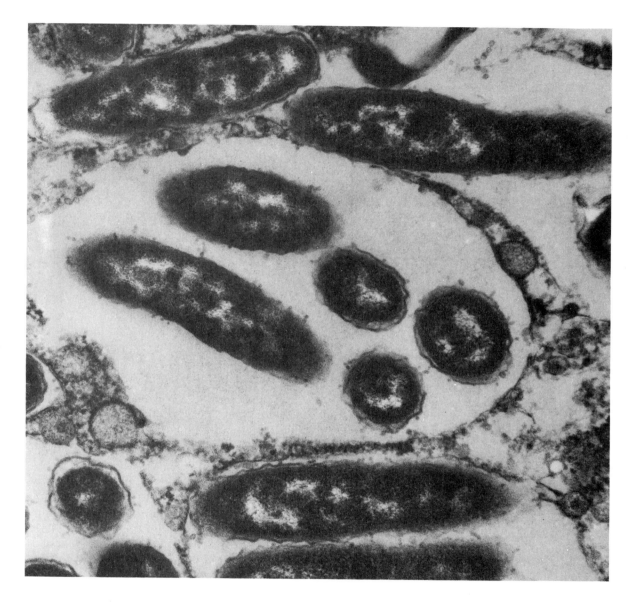

Figure 2.6 LEGIONELLA PNEUMOPHILIA is stained with uranyl acetate and lead citrate and enlarged some 45,000 diameters in an electron micrograph of the yolk sac from an infected embryonated egg. The organism, seen in longitudinal and transverse sections, is structurally similar to some other bacteria but appears to be unrelated to any previously described species or genus; hence the name *L. pneumophilia.*

mission their condition deteriorates. In the absence of specific treatment about 20 percent of these patients die of progressive pneumonia (which interferes with the oxygenation of the blood) or from shock (the mechanism of which is not known, but which may result from the presence of bacteria in the blood). The other 80 percent recover gradually over a week or more, during which time some of them may require mechanical help in breathing or dialysis to deal with kidney failure. Recovery is usu-

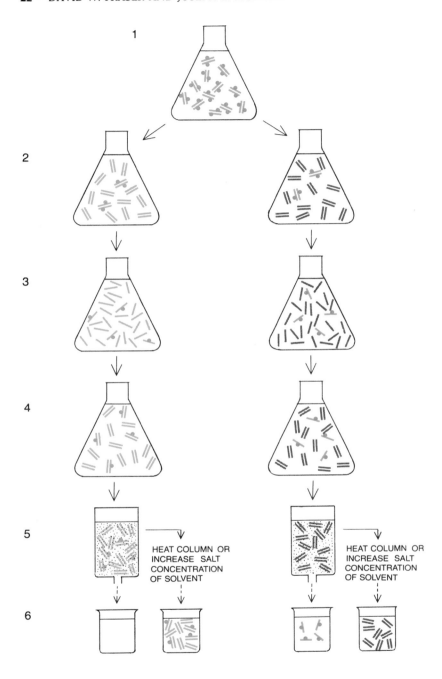

Figure 2.7 DNA-HYBRIDIZATION TEST. Double-strand DNA of *L. pneumophilia* (*light color*) is labeled with a radioactive isotope (*color dot*) and broken into short lengths (*1*). Labeled DNA is mixed with short pieces of unlabeled DNA (*2*) from the same bacterium (*left*) and from another bacterium (*gray*) being tested for relatedness (*right*). The mixtures are heated, forming single strands of DNA (*3*), then cooled and incubated; complementary strands collide and reassociate (*4*). The labeled DNA pieces mixed with homologous DNA "find" a complementary unlabeled strand (*left*), but the labeled DNA pieces mixed with DNA from a different bacterium do not (*right*). The single- and double-strand DNA's are separated (*5*) and collected (*6*).

HEAT COLUMN OR INCREASE SALT CONCENTRATION OF SOLVENT

HEAT COLUMN OR INCREASE SALT CONCENTRATION OF SOLVENT

ally complete, although patients may feel weak for several months and there may be a certain amount of permanent lung damage.

Pontiac fever begins much as Legionnaires' disease does, with headache, muscle aches and fever, but typically the symptoms appear only a day or two after exposure. Symptoms include coughing, chest pain, diarrhea, vomiting, sore throat and confusion, but ordinarily these symptoms are not prominent. Neither pneumonia nor shock has been seen in Pontiac fever, nor have the kidneys or the liver been involved. Patients have fever and feel

	LEGIONNAIRES' DISEASE	PONTIAC FEVER
ATTACK RATE	1 – 5 PERCENT	95 PERCENT
INCUBATION PERIOD	TWO TO 10 DAYS	ONE TO TWO DAYS
SYMPTOMS	FEVER, COUGH, MUSCLE ACHES, CHILLS, HEADACHE, CHEST PAIN, SPUTUM, DIARRHEA, CONFUSION	FEVER, COUGH, MUSCLE ACHES, CHILLS, HEADACHE, CHEST PAIN, CONFUSION
EFFECTS ON LUNG	PNEUMONIA, PLEURAL EFFUSION	PLEURITIS, NO PNEUMONIA
OTHER AFFECTED ORGAN SYSTEMS	KIDNEY, LIVER, GASTROINTESTINAL TRACT, NERVOUS SYSTEM	NONE
CASE-FATALITY RATIO	15– 20 PERCENT	NO FATALITIES

Figure 2.8 LEGIONELLOSIS (disease caused by *L. pneumophila*) has been seen in two basic forms: Legionnaires' disease and Pontiac fever. The major distinguishing features are the attack rate (much higher in Pontiac fever), the incubation period (shorter in Pontiac fever) and the presence of pneumonia in Legionnaires' disease but not in Pontiac fever, a much milder illness.

very sick for from two to five days, but they all recover, apparently completely.

It is still not clear which antibiotics are most effective in *L. pneumophila* infections; no randomized trials with controls have been done with human beings. Claire V. Broome and her colleagues at the CDC did observe that during a 1977 epidemic in Vermont only one person of 22 who were treated with erythromycin died, whereas 10 of 41 who did not receive erythromycin died. Clyde Thornsberry found that growth of the bacterium on agar is inhibited by rather low concentrations of several antibiotics, but the organism manufactures an enzyme that inactivates most antibiotics of one group, the cephalosporins. Infected chick embryos were best protected by erythromycin, rifampin, gentamicin, streptomycin, sulfadiazine or chloramphenicol. With Theodore F. Tsai and others we found that infected guinea pigs recovered after treatment with erythromycin or rifampin. At this stage physicians are advised to treat patients who may have Legionnaires' disease with erythromycin, with rifampin therapy added for those who do not respond. Antibiotic therapy is apparently not required for Pontiac fever.

DIAGNOSIS

The clinical features that help to distinguish Legionnaires' disease from other pneumonias include diarrhea, confusion, lack of runny nose or sore throat, red blood cells in the urine, abnormalities of liver function, absence of the usual pneumonia-causing bacteria in the sputum and, of course, the failure to respond to courses of treatment that have been shown to be ineffective against *L. pneumophila*.

A specific diagnosis of legionellosis can be made only by isolating the organism from the patient, by showing a rise in the level of antibodies to the bacterium as the patient recovers or by demonstrating the presence of *L. pneumophila* itself in the patient's tissues or body fluids. The organism has been isolated from blood, sputum, pleural fluid and lung tissue by the inoculation of either guinea pigs or the appropriate bacteriologic mediums. There are practical limitations, however, on attempts to isolate the bacterium directly on a culture medium. It can be hard to obtain suitable specimens, the organism is not readily cultured and it takes several days for the cultured bacterium to grow.

By means of the indirect fluorescent-antibody technique high concentrations of antibody can be demonstrated by the end of the second week of illness in about half of the patients tested, but some patients do not develop antibodies until the sixth week and about 15 percent of them never achieve significant levels. There are other techniques for demonstrating antibodies, but their sensitivity and specificity are not well established. Another problem is that there are several different serologic groups of *L. pneumophila,* each one carrying a different set of antigens. An infection may be caused by a member of any group, so that the patient's serum must be tested against representatives of each group. Moreover, a diagnosis based on a rise in the level of antibodies to the organism must necessarily be retrospective. It is usually only during convalescence that the antibody level is high enough to be firmly diagnostic, and that is obviously too late to help the physician choose the right therapy.

Direct fluorescent-antibody testing, on the other hand, can make diagnosis possible within a few hours, early in the course of infection. The patient's sputum or other respiratory secretion is exposed to antibodies to *L. pneumophila* (prepared by immunizing rabbits with inactivated bacteria) that have been conjugated to a fluorescent material. The antibodies become fixed to the *L. pneumophila* antigens, revealing the presence of the bacterium. As many as 70 percent of the patients may show positive fluorescent staining, and false-positive results seem to be infrequent. Preliminary work suggests that antigens of the organism can be detected in patient's serum and urine by a sophisticated procedure called enzyme-linked immunosorbence. If this test proves to be sufficiently sensitive and specific, it should be of great value in making early diagnoses.

OCCURRENCE OF THE DISEASE

In the few years since legionellosis was recognized as a new disease entity cases have been discovered almost wherever they were sought: in more than 40 states of the U.S. and also in Australia, Canada, Denmark, Greece, Israel, Italy, the Netherlands, Norway, Spain, Sweden, Switzerland, West Germany, the United Kingdom and Yugoslavia. No significant geographical pattern has yet emerged, but information from many regions of the world is still lacking or is sketchy. Sometimes there are clusters of cases that appear to have a common source and sometimes there are isolated single cases; almost all the clusters and most of the sporadic cases have been reported in the summer.

Legionnaires' disease is most often seen in middle-aged and elderly people, although children as young as 16 months have been affected. More men are affected than women. The disease is commoner in cigarette smokers (but not in cigar or pipe smokers) and in heavy drinkers. Underlying medical problems, such as cancer, leukemia, lymphoma and kidney failure, and drugs that impair the immune system appear to predispose a person to Legionnaires' disease (and to other infections).

Gregory A. Storch and William B. Baine of the CDC have found that sporadic cases are more frequent among travelers, construction workers and people living near sites of excavation or construction. It may be that such people are more likely to be exposed to airborne dust, which may carry the bacteria. Outbreaks of legionellosis have usually been concentrated in or near a building, often a hotel or a hospital. In some instances the building appears to have been simply a place where large numbers of susceptible people congregated, but in other instances the central air-conditioning system has been implicated as the source of the bacteria (for reasons that will be made clear below).

The overall incidence of legionellosis is not known with precision. When Hjordis M. Foy of the University of Washington School of Public Health and her co-workers did a prospective study of pneumonia among people enrolled in a health program, their results indicated that *L. pneumophila* was the cause of 12 cases per 100,000 of population per year. If this rate applies nationwide, there are some 26,000 cases of legionellosis in the U.S. per year. Between .3 and 1.5 percent of the serum specimens from pneumonia patients submitted to the CDC have shown evidence of legionellosis. If those specimens are broadly representative of all pneumonia patients, from 7,000 to 36,000 of the nation's 2.4 million annual cases of pneumonia are in fact cases of Legionnaires' disease.

ECOLOGY OF THE DISEASE

Most infectious agents that cause epidemics of pneumonia but do not spread from person to person are found to spread through the air from some characteristic ecological niche in the nonhuman environment. A common example is the fungus *Histoplasma capsulatum,* which lives in the soil and causes disease when contaminated dust is stirred up and inhaled. It seemed likely that *L. pneumophila* might live in such an inanimate environment; this hypothesis was strengthened by laboratory studies showing that the bacterium could survive (although apparently not proliferate) for more than a year in tap water.

The 1965 outbreak at St. Elizabeth's Hospital suggested that *L. pneumophila* might live in the soil. During the summer of that epidemic several sites on the hospital grounds had been excavated for the installation of a new lawn-sprinkler system. Stephen B. Thacker and John V. Bennett of the CDC found that it was mainly patients whose beds were near windows in buildings close to excavation sites who became ill. The cases were clustered in time, with each cluster coming five or six days after an excavation site had been filled in, suggesting that contaminated dust raised in the process had spread through the air to infect the patients. No attempt was made in 1965 to recover a disease agent from the soil (and, as we have shown, it would have been difficult to isolate *L. pneumophila* from such specimens in any case), but the organism has since been isolated from mud at other locations.

In three recorded outbreaks the water in the cooling towers or evaporative condensers of air-conditioning systems has been implicated as the source of infection (see Figure 2.9). In a cooling tower the water that has been warmed by heat from a compressor is sprayed over splash bars of wood or other material as air is drawn past the falling droplets by a fan. Some of the water evaporates, cooling the rest, which is recirculated. A small amount of water is entrained as drift, or minute droplets in the exhausted air; the drift carries with it whatever is in the cooling-tower water, including any bacteria that may be present, and it can be carried a considerable distance. In an evaporative condenser the water is

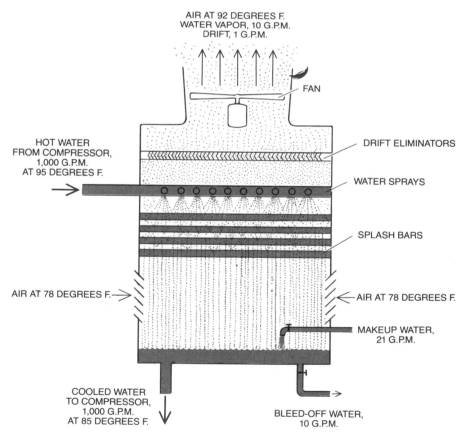

Figure 2.9 COOLING TOWERS for air-conditioning systems have been implicated as spreaders of *L. pneumophila*. A typical cooling tower of a size appropriate for a hotel, hospital or large office building may handle about 1,000 gallons of water per minute. Coolant water from the compressor is sprayed over splash bars; a fan draws fresh air through the spray to maximize evaporation, which cools the water. Some water is exhausted as vapor and a small amount of drift (water droplets); the rest is recirculated. Airborne bacteria could be drawn in by fan, entrained in spray water and exhausted in drift. In one case drift from tower contaminated conditioned air.

sprayed over metal coils containing the refrigerant, which is cooled directly by the evaporation of the water.

In two outbreaks associated with evaporative condensers and one associated with a cooling tower, patients were shown to have been exposed to drift. In all three instances L. pneumophila was isolated from water found in the cooling device. George K. Morris of the CDC has also recovered the bacterium from towers that are not known to have been associated with any cases of legionellosis, and it therefore seems likely that both the towers and the condensers are quite commonly contaminated with airborne soil bacteria gathered from the air by the spraying water. If this is the case, the conditions remain to be defined under which certain towers and condensers that are contaminated but for a time do no harm come to disseminate the bacteria. Meanwhile studies are under way to find antibacterial agents that are effective against L. pneumophila and could serve to decontaminate air-conditioning equipment.

UNANSWERED QUESTIONS

It seems paradoxical that an organism so fastidious in its nutritional requirements and so hard to grow in the laboratory apparently persists and succeeds so well in an inanimate environment. L. pneumophila's precise ecological niche and nutritional supply have not been defined. Learning its natural history would be a big step toward understanding how people are exposed to the bacterium in individual cases of legionellosis and under what conditions outbreaks develop.

It is still not known why L. pneumophila causes two such different illnesses as Legionnaires' disease and Pontiac fever, or why the bacterium affects only 1 percent of the people apparently exposed to it in the case of the former illness and as many as 95 percent in the case of the latter one. It may be that strains of the bacterium differ in some critical way that determines which illness develops. Laboratory testing, including a search for toxins secreted by the bacterium, has yet, however, to show any significant difference between the Pontiac strain and the Philadelphia one.

It is quite possible that Legionnaires' disease and Pontiac fever are not the only disease syndromes caused by L. pneumophila. Clinicians have only recently begun to investigate the possibility that the bacterium may be responsible, for example, for certain cases of lung abscess and endocarditis (inflammation of the lining of the heart). Moreover, only about two-thirds of the 2.4 million annual U.S. pneumonia cases can be linked to a known viral or bacterial agent; what causes the 800,000 or so other cases is not known, and identifying the agents is currently a major challenge. It is conceivable that some of the unknown agents are bacteria related to L. pneumophila that have not yet been detected. Continuing investigation of legionellosis should provide an opportunity to find any such related organisms.

POSTSCRIPT

Our discussion has turned from one of the most ancient diseases, plague, to one of the most modern, legionellosis. Is it really possible that despite the intense effort of thousands of scientists and doctors over the past century, new infectious diseases are still being discovered? Epidemiologic research has often been likened to detective work, and the story of Legionnaires' disease illustrates this well. The quick solution to the deaths at the Bellevue-Stratford Hotel in Philadelphia attests to the expert brilliance of our medical detectives at the CDC in Atlanta, Georgia. Within a year of the first outbreak of legionellosis, these public servants, toiling tirelessly, had not only discovered the cause, but had found a cure.

Although the bacterium that causes legionellosis is not especially difficult to culture, at the beginning the researchers had no idea what the organism was like. They thus had to employ the most general type of culture medium, a living organism. Parasites that are incapable of growth in nonliving culture media are called obligate parasites and for many years chick embryos have been used in research on such obligate parasites as viruses and rickettsia. It was thus natural to use this widely available host to search for the Legionnaires' disease pathogen. Once positive results had been obtained in the chick embryo, microscopic procedures and staining methods could be used to discover what the causal organism looked like. After the organism was spotted, it was determined that it was an ordinary bacterium (albeit of a new type), and it was then relatively easy to develop a nonliving culture medium in which the organism could be grown for further study.

Immunology played a major role in the study of legionellosis, as it does in most modern research on infectious diseases. Once the causal bacterium was available in culture, it was possible to use the bacterium as an antigen to search for antibodies in patients or their contacts. With the reasonable assumption that the presence of an antibody against the bacterium indicates present or earlier infection, it was possible to trace the spread of epidemics of legionellosis through suspected human populations.

Legionellosis seems to occur primarily in people whose immune system is less vigorous. Elderly people, those who smoke or drink heavily, and those who suffer from underlying medical problems, are more likely to succumb to legionellosis (as well as to other infections).

One of the great breakthroughs in understanding the ecology of the disease was the discovery that the disease was associated in some way with cooling towers and air-conditioning units. This suggested that the bacterium might actually have its primary habitat in such structures and reach humans only accidentally in mists and droplets. Thus, one way to reduce the incidence of legionellosis is to treat cooling towers and air-conditioning units from time to time with disinfectants.

Another surprising location for legionellosis has been discovered since the early work reported here: nursing homes. Nursing home patients often have, of course, impaired immune systems, so they are definitely at risk for legionellosis. But where does the bacterium come from? The organism actually lives in the hot-water tanks of the nursing homes and reaches human lungs by way of the mists that occur when showers are taken. The bacterium *Legionella pneumophila* is surprisingly tolerant to higher temperatures and may actually grow in hot-water tanks. Interestingly, the energy crisis of the 1970's actually increased the likelihood of *Legionella* infection by way of hot water, since to save energy costs the temperatures of many hot-water heaters were lowered, making them more favorable for the growth of *L. pneumophila*. Of course, *L. pneumophila* grows in all hot-water heaters of the appropriate temperature, not just those of nursing homes, but because the patients in nursing homes are more likely to be susceptible to legionellosis, outbreaks occur there more readily.

A historical note: The Bellevue-Stratford Hotel, once the jewel of Philadelphia society, was at the time of the 1976 Legionnaires' convention an aging structure that was barely making a profit. As a result of the unfavorable publicity resulting from the outbreak of legionellosis, it was forced to close its doors and go out of business. However, it later was completely refurbished (the offending air-conditioning unit was removed), and the hotel is now finding its rightful place in the commercial and convention life of the City of Brotherly Love.

Lyme Disease

A bacterium transmitted to human beings by the bite of a deer tick causes this hazard of summertime. Interleukin-1, an immune-system regulator, may mediate its potentially serious arthritis-like symptoms.

. . .

Gail S. Habicht, Gregory Beck and Jorge L. Benach
July, 1987

Lyme disease is an affliction of summer. It is a tickborne bacterial disease that is most likely to be contracted during the months of June through September, when youngsters and adults are outdoors, walking barelegged in woods and long grass.

It is spreading rapidly and is now the most frequently diagnosed tick-transmitted illness in the U.S., if not in the world. In 1975, 59 cases were recorded in Connecticut; in 1985 the number had climbed to 863 cases. Moreover, Lyme disease has now spread to three regions of the U.S. (see Figure 3.1): the Northeast (in coastal areas), the northern Middle West (Minnesota and Wisconsin) and the West (parts of California, Oregon, Utah and Nevada). The disease is also found throughout Europe and has been recorded in Australia, the Soviet Union, China, Japan and Africa.

Because its symptoms can be severe, ranging from acute headache to neurological impairment and manifestations resembling rheumatoid arthritis, the disease has elicited concern in the 12 years since it was first described. The discovery of this disease, from its recognition as a clinical entity to the identification of its causative agent, is a triumph of modern medical research and a tribute to the collaborative efforts of a great many scientists.

Lyme disease was first reported in November of 1975, when the Connecticut State Health Department received telephone calls from two mothers whose children had just been diagnosed as having juvenile rheumatoid arthritis. The condition is a devastating one that can lead to lifelong suffering and physical debilitation, and it is not surprising that these mothers were concerned. What alarmed Health Department officials, however, was the news that these cases were not isolated ones: according to the women who telephoned, a number of adults and children in the town of Lyme had recently been diagnosed as having rheumatoid arthritis. Health officials concluded that this was more than a regional anomaly and might represent something very serious: either the presence of an environmental toxin or possibly the beginning of an epidemic.

They contacted Allen C. Steere, who was then a postdoctoral fellow in rheumatology at the Yale University School of Medicine. He had just completed training with the epidemic-intelligence ser-

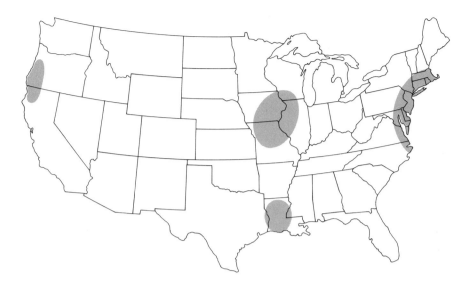

Figure 3.1 LYME DISEASE continues to spread throughout the U.S.; it has been reported in 25 states. Most cases are found along the North Atlantic coast from Massachusetts to North Carolina, in Minnesota and Wisconsin, in Texas and along the Pacific coast in California and Oregon. Scattered cases, however, have also been reported from Arkansas, Florida, Georgia, Indiana, Kentucky, Maine, Michigan, Montana, Nevada, New Hampshire, Ohio, Tennessee, Utah and Vermont. The areas of heaviest incidence are indicated in color.

vice of the U.S. Centers for Disease Control in Atlanta. Intrigued by this bizarre outbreak of arthritis, he agreed to undertake an epidemiological investigation.

Steere and his colleagues discovered that the disease was limited to three townships in eastern Connecticut, Old Lyme, Lyme and East Haddam, which are adjacent communities on the east bank of the Connecticut River. Juvenile rheumatoid arthritis is normally a rare condition, affecting only one in 100,000 children, and yet out of a total population of 12,000 in these three towns, 39 children (and 12 adults) had been diagnosed as having the condition: 100 times the normal occurrence.

Moreover, distinct cluster patterns emerged within each town. Most victims lived in heavily wooded areas and only a few of them in town centers. In Old Lyme and East Haddam half of the affected individuals lived on just four roads, and here the frequency in children was 10,000 times higher than normal: one in 10 children as opposed to an expected one in 100,000. This was clearly no ordinary form of rheumatoid arthritis, and there were few clues to guide Steere in his investigation. Nevertheless, he made several important findings.

One was that the disease is not particularly contagious: individuals in the same family often contracted it in different years. Another was that the majority of cases, regardless of the year, first presented symptoms during the summer months, June through September. A third finding was that 25 percent of the patients Steere interviewed remembered having a strange skin rash from one to several weeks before the onset of arthritis-like symptoms. The descriptions of the rashes were remarkably similar: they had started as a red papule, or small bump, and gradually expanded to form a bull's-eye from 10 to 50 centimeters in diameter. The occurrence of the rash on the chest, abdomen, back or buttocks of most patients suggested that most likely a crawling, rather than a flying, insect or an arachnid had transmitted the disease, although no one could clearly remember being bitten.

Steere concluded on the basis of these findings that he was dealing with a previously unrecognized disease probably caused by a virus and transmitted by an unknown arthropod (the group to which insects, spiders and ticks belong). He named it Lyme arthritis or Lyme disease for the town in which it was first observed. In 1975–76 he began testing sera from victims of Lyme disease for the presence of specific antibodies against 38 known tick-transmitted diseases and 178 other arthropod-transmitted viruses. Not a single test result was positive.

As he carried out research on the disease and its probable causes, however, Steere came across some interesting information. In 1909 a similar phenomenon had been described in Europe. A Swedish physician, Arvid Afzelius, described an expanding red skin rash in patients who had been bitten by the tick *Ixodes ricinus*. Afzelius named the rash erythema chronicum migrans (ECM), which literally means "chronic migrating red rash."

ECM sounded remarkably like the bull's-eye rash that had been observed in Lyme disease patients. Although it lacked the arthritis-like symptoms characteristic of Lyme disease, Steere concluded that ECM and Lyme disease might be closely related and have similar modes of transmission.

European physicians had successfully treated ECM with penicillin, indicating that the most likely agent of infection was not a virus but a bacterium. Yet when fluid was removed from the joints of Lyme disease patients and cultured, no microorganisms could be found. Meanwhile the number of cases of Lyme disease continued to climb.

Finally, in 1977, nine patients affected by the ECM rash that year remembered having been bitten by a tick at the site of the rash. One of them had removed the tick and saved it, and was able to give it to Steere for identification. The tick, barely larger than a pinhead, was a dark brown, hard-bodied animal that might easily be mistaken for a scab or a piece of dirt. It was not surprising that it had taken Steere and his group almost two years to locate it.

The tick was identified by Andrew Spielman of the Harvard School of Public Health as *Ixodes dammini* (see Figure 3.2), a species closely related to *I. ricinus*, the tick responsible for European ECM. Now that *I. dammini* was identified, investigators working on Lyme disease hoped to isolate the actual agent of infection. First they had to be certain that the tick was indeed the vector for Lyme disease. If the distribution of *I. dammini* in the wild corresponded to the outbreak of Lyme disease, the circumstantial evidence linking the two would be strong indeed.

Biologists at Yale set out animal traps on both sides of the Connecticut River in order to map the distribution of *Ixodes* along the river and at the same time find out on which mammalian species it was feeding. The distribution of ticks was just as they hoped: the dog tick *Dermacentor variabilis* was equally common on both sides of the river, but *I. dammini* was 12 times more abundant on the east side — near Lyme, Old Lyme and East Haddam, where Lyme disease was by that time known to be endemic. The workers were convinced that *I. dammini* must be the primary vector in the transmission of Lyme disease.

Still the agent responsible for both ECM and Lyme disease remained elusive. Repeated cell cultures and microscopic examinations of the tick's internal organs failed to reveal the presence of a bacterium or any other pathogen. Then, in the fall of 1981, a fatal case of Rocky Mountain spotted fever, a rickettsial disease transmitted by the dog tick, was reported on Shelter Island, off the coast of eastern Long Island. The New York State Department of Health sent a team of biologists to the island to collect live ticks. Because the normal vector, *Dermacentor variabilis*, is not found in the fall, adult *Ixodes dammini* were collected instead and were sent to the Rocky Mountain Laboratories in Hamilton, Mont., for study.

There Willy Burgdorfer, an international authority on tickborne diseases, squashed the digestive tract of the *Ixodes* tick and examined it by dark-field microscopy. To his surprise he found the gut teeming not with the rickettsiae that cause Rocky Mountain spotted fever but with long, irregularly shaped spirochete bacteria. Burgdorfer knew that *I. dammini* had been implicated as the probable vector for Lyme disease, and he also knew that the spirochetes were not the infectious agent of Rocky Mountain spotted fever. He wondered whether these bacteria could be the cause of Lyme disease. Fortunately Alan G. Barbour, then at the Rocky Mountain Laboratories, was able to grow the spirochetes in pure culture and obtain them in sufficient quantities for experimentation.

Because patients exposed to an infectious agent have antibodies in their serum that react to the agent, an antibody test can be a good indicator of infection. Serum samples from New York patients infected with Lyme disease were sent to Burgdorfer, who tested them for the presence of antibodies against the spirochetes. Unlike the earlier series of tests conducted by Steere, the results this time were positive: the sera showed a pronounced antibody

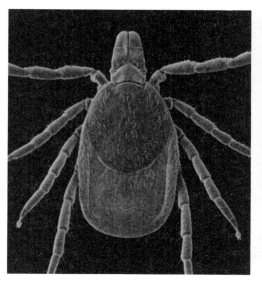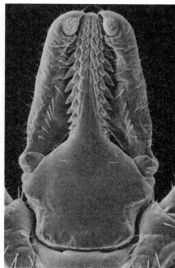

Figure 3.2 SCANNING ELECTRON MICROGRAPHS of a female *I. dammini* show the animal, enlarged 26 diameters, in dorsal view (*left*) and a close-up of the head, enlarged 120 diameters, in ventral view (*right*). The legs have claws and adhesive pads at their tips that help the tick cling to its host while feeding. The head consists of a small cranium and a large proboscis, called the hypostome, surrounded by sensory palps. The hypostome drills through the skin of a host until it reaches a capillary and then draws blood out of the host and into the tick. The serrations on the hypostome's surface help to anchor it in place once it has pierced a blood vessel. (Photos by S. F. Hayes, W. Burgdorfer and M. D. Corwin at the Rocky Mountain Laboratories.)

response to the bacteria, indicating that the patients had in fact been infected by the spirochete.

A more direct test of the pathogenicity of the spirochete was carried out on rabbits. Spirochete-infected ticks were placed on the shaved skin of albino rabbits, where they could be observed feeding on the blood of their hosts. After several weeks lesions similar to the ECM rash appeared, and microscopic examination of the skin at the site of tick attachment revealed the presence of live spirochetes.

From this point investigations proceeded rapidly. By the summer of 1982 spirochetes had been isolated from the blood, skin and cerebrospinal fluid of Lyme disease victims by investigators at the New York State Department of Health and at Yale. Russell C. Johnson and his colleagues at the University of Minnesota Medical School studied the Lyme disease spirochete and determined, on the basis of its DNA, that it was a new species in the genus *Borrelia*. In 1984, to honor its discoverer, Burgdorfer, they named it *Borrelia burgdorferi*.

B. burgdorferi is a typical spirochete: it is a unicel-lular, loosely coiled, left-handed helix (that is, it coils in a counterclockwise direction). Its length varies but averages 30 micrometers (thousandths of a millimeter), with seven turns of the coil. Like most spirochetes, it is small and difficult to detect: the diameter of the cell ranges from .18 to .25 micrometer, allowing it to pass through many filters designed to retain bacteria.

Once *B. burgdorferi* had been conclusively identified as the agent of Lyme disease it was possible to track its distribution in nature. Edward M. Bosler of the New York State Department of Health found the spirochete in the tissues of several mammals, including field mice, voles and deer, as well as in all stages of *I. dammini* (see Figure 3.3).

Detection of the spirochete in mammalian tissue is difficult. Not only is the spirochete extremely small but also it is normally present in very low numbers. The preferred method of detection therefore depends on fluorescein-labeled antibodies specific for *B. burgdorferi*. These bind to the spirochetes and fluoresce on illumination with ultraviolet light, making it possible to detect the presence of even a few spirochetes. Such studies indicate that *Borrelia*

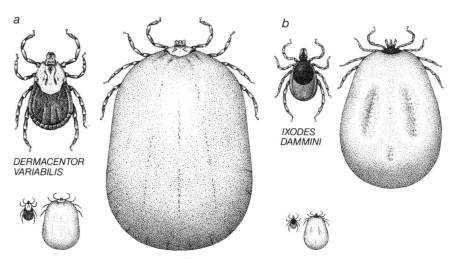

Figure 3.3 COMMON DISEASE-CARRYING ticks in the U.S. are the dog tick *Dermacentor variabilis* (*a*), which transmits the bacterium that causes Rocky Mountain spotted fever, and the deer tick *Ixodes dammini* (*b*), which transmits the Lyme disease spirochete. Both tick species feed on the blood of mammalian hosts, including human beings, and may triple in size following a meal. The bottom drawings show the actual size of each tick species and compare ticks that have not fed recently (*left*) with ticks that are engorged by a meal (*right*). The top drawings (enlarged four times) show greater anatomical detail.

travels widely once it enters the bloodstream: it has been detected in the eyes, kidneys, spleen, liver, testes and brain of nonhuman mammalian hosts, and also in several species of passerine birds. (The geographic distribution of Lyme disease suggests that *Borrelia* spreads when ticks infested with the bacterium attach themselves to migratory birds.)

Borrelia burgdorferi can be detected in the gut of *I. dammini* by dark-field microscopy or by removing the contents of the tick's gut and growing the spirochetes in culture. Surveys along the North Atlantic coastline indicate that in highly endemic areas from 80 to 90 percent of *Ixodes* ticks have *B. burgdorferi* in their gastrointestinal systems. In contrast, only 3 percent of all *Ixodes* tested on the West Coast harbor the spirochete, a finding that correlates well with the much lower incidence of Lyme disease there.

The life cycle of *I. dammini* normally spans two years (see Figure 3.4). Eggs are deposited in the spring and hatch into free-living larvae a month later. During the first summer the larva feeds once (for a period of two days) on the blood of a host and then enters a resting stage coincident with the onset of cold weather in the fall. The following spring the larva molts, enters a second immature stage called the nymphal stage and again attaches itself to an animal host, this time to feed for three or four days.

Although the larvae and nymphs attack a variety of vertebrates, the majority of the ticks in these age cohorts are found on the white-footed mouse, *Peromyscus leucopus*. It is at this stage that ticks are most likely to attach themselves to humans.

At the end of the summer nymphs molt into the adult stage. They can be found in brush about one meter above the ground, where they can easily attach themselves to larger mammals. Like the immature ticks, the adults feed on a variety of mammalian hosts, but in the northeastern U.S. they are found predominately on the white-tailed deer, *Odocoileus virginianus*. The adult ticks mate on the host soon after the female attaches herself to it. Only the females overwinter; the males die soon after mating. It is not known where the eggs are deposited, but they hatch in the spring—and the entire cycle is repeated.

Anyone who lives in or visits an area where Lyme disease is endemic is susceptible to the condition. Warning signs have been posted in areas where the infestation is particularly high (see Figure 3.5). Lyme disease is indiscriminate: it affects both sexes and all age groups. Although disproportionate numbers of children have been affected, this may simply reflect the fact that children spend more time playing in wooded areas than adults do. In addition, people who have outdoor animals are known to be

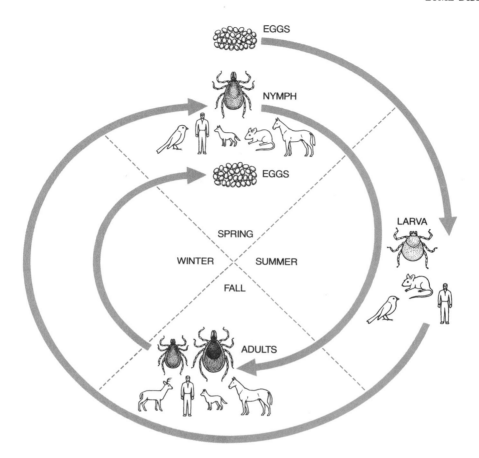

Figure 3.4 LIFE CYCLE of *I. dammini* lasts for two years. Eggs are deposited in the spring and the larvae (which have only six legs) emerge several weeks later. They feed once during the summer, usually on the blood of small mammals such as mice. Larvae molt the following spring into slightly larger eight-legged nymphs, which also feed once during the summer—on mice or larger mammals such as dogs, deer or human beings—before molting into adults in the fall. Adults attach themselves to a host, usually the white-tailed deer, where they mate. The males die shortly thereafter, but the females continue to feed to obtain the protein necessary for egg development. Females lay their eggs and die.

at greater risk for contracting Lyme disease, but it is not clear whether this reflects a more outdoor lifestyle or the fact that the humans are bitten by ticks attached to the fur of their domestic animals. Lyme disease is also rapidly becoming a veterinary problem: dogs and horses in endemic areas have developed debilitating joint problems that veterinarians believe are caused by *Borrelia burgdorferi*.

Clinically Lyme disease can be divided into three stages. The first and most obvious stage is characterized by the erythema chronicum migrans rash (see Figure 3.6), which develops from two to 30 days after an individual has been bitten. The rash is frequently accompanied by profound fatigue, fever, chills, headache and backache. In some patients, however, these symptoms, including ECM, fail to appear. In from 25 to 50 percent of cases secondary lesions appear at various sites on the body. Because these lack distinct red papules at their center, they probably reflect the spreading of spirochetes by way of the blood, rather than additional tick bites.

The second stage (also not always expressed) is marked by neurological complications and migratory musculoskeletal pain. Approximately 5 percent of patients develop cardiac difficulties lasting for from three days to six weeks. These patients experience palpitations, dizziness or shortness of breath

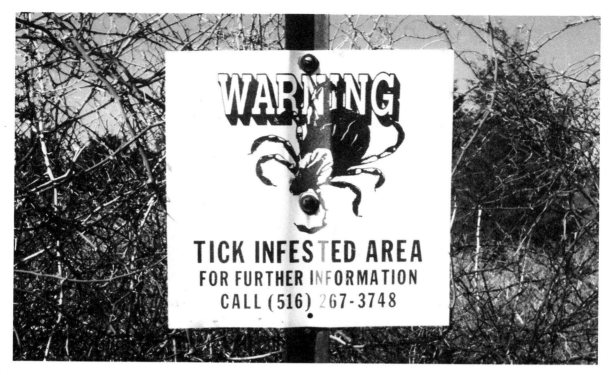

Figure 3.5 HEALTH WARNING posted near the Atlantic coast in Amagansett, N.Y., is one of many such notices distributed throughout tick-infested areas on Long Island. Lyme disease is rapidly increasing in wooded areas where the mammals on which the ticks feed are abundant. People who develop symptoms characteristic of Lyme disease are advised to seek prompt treatment from a physician.

associated with irregular electrical impulses to the heart (atrioventricular block), and some may require temporary pacemakers.

The third stage typically involves the onset of arthritis. Joint problems characteristic of rheumatoid arthritis occur in about 60 percent of Lyme disease patients who have not been treated, generally within several months but not more than two years after the onset of ECM. Attacks of arthritis usually last from a few days to a few weeks at a time and primarily affect the knees (which can lead to difficulty in walking) and other large joints.

The nervous system may be involved in all stages of Lyme disease: live spirochetes have been detected in the cerebrospinal fluid and brain tissue of patients diagnosed as having the disease. The episodic, excruciating headaches and neck pain experienced during the first stage are believed to result from irritation of the meninges, the membranes surrounding the brain. During the second stage 15 percent of patients develop more severe neurological complications, including meningitis, inflamed nerve roots in the neck and Bell's palsy: a paralysis of the seventh cranial nerve, which controls many facial muscles. Some patients experience increased sensitivity of the skin to touch or changes in temperature. During the third stage a small percentage of patients also suffer from somnolence, loss of memory, mood swings and an inability to concentrate.

Fortunately Lyme disease can be treated successfully at any stage with broad-spectrum antibiotics administered orally, including penicillin, tetracycline and erythromycin. Current studies suggest that cephalosporin antibiotics are also effective. Treatment during the first stage greatly reduces the likelihood of developing neurological, cardiac or arthritic complications. Even if it is left untreated until the third stage, Lyme disease can still be eradicated

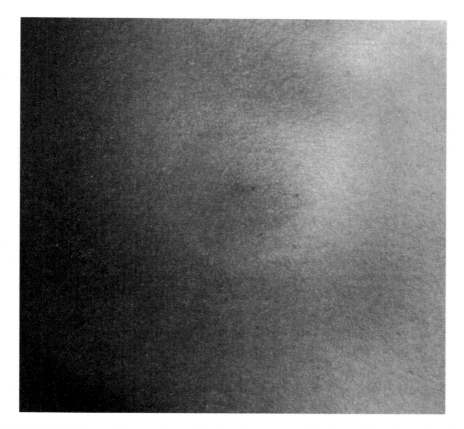

Figure 3.6 FIRST STAGE of Lyme disease, observed in 60 percent of the individuals bitten by infected *Ixodes* ticks, is very pronounced. It appears as a large bull's-eye rash, which expands radially from the site of the tick bite (seen here as a small red papule) and is noticeably swollen at its center. The rash on this patient's back measures 14 centimeters in diameter. (Photograph provided by the New York State Department of Health.)

in most patients by antibiotic therapy, although hospitalization and intravenous administration of the antibiotics may be necessary at this stage.

Physicians who treat patients with Lyme disease have observed an unusual phenomenon. Immediately following antibiotic therapy there is a temporary exacerbation of symptoms. This phenomenon, known as the Jarisch-Herxheimer reaction, was first seen in syphilis patients who were treated with mercury ointments in the 16th century. Syphilis is also caused by a spirochete, *Treponema pallidum*, and it shares many symptoms with Lyme disease including rashes, joint involvement and neurological complications. The Jarisch-Herxheimer reaction has also been observed following treatment of other spirochete infections, such as relapsing fever. The reac-

tion has given us a major clue for elucidating the pathogenesis of Lyme disease.

It is interesting that Lyme disease patients experience an extensive array of symptoms in spite of the presence of only a small number of spirochetes. Two theories of Lyme disease pathogenesis have been advanced to explain this fact; both involve the immune system and both appear to be operative. The first theory holds that immune complexes, which consist of antigens from the spirochete and antibodies and complement from the human host, accumulate in a patient's joints. This buildup in turn attracts neutrophils (phagocytic white blood cells), which release a variety of enzymes that attack the antigen-antibody complexes. According to this hypothesis, it is the enzymes released by the neutrophils that attack the joint and erode bone and cartilage tissue to cause arthritis-like symptoms.

Work done in our laboratory at the State University of New York at Stony Brook suggests a second hypothesis. We believe the pathological effects of spirochetes are amplified not only by neutrophil-secreted enzymes but also by the immune-system mediator called interleukin-1 (IL-1) (see Figure 3.7).

IL-1 is a protein with a molecular weight of 17,000 daltons that is synthesized primarily by the phagocytic white blood cells called macrophages. It is a regulator of the body's immune response and acts as the molecular orchestrator of nonspecific defense mechanisms against a variety of environmental insults. It coordinates the body's reaction to bacterial infection and trauma by regulating the onset of fever, the release of neutrophils from bone marrow and the proliferation of fibroblasts (connective-tissue cells).

One of the most powerful stimuli for the release of IL-1 is a lipopolysaccharide (LPS), a complex of sugar and lipid molecules, that is found in the outer envelope of the cell wall of all gram-negative bacteria. Because Borrelia burgdorferi is a gram-negative bacterium, we speculated that it might contain LPS

that could trigger the release of IL-1, which in turn would exert powerful local and systemic effects on the human body.

We approached our hypothesis in several ways. First we needed to demonstrate that the cell wall of B. burgdorferi does indeed contain LPS. To do this we cultured the spirochetes in a special growth medium and then harvested large numbers of them, which we tested for the presence of LPS. Once we confirmed that LPS was present, we applied a chemical extraction method to isolate the LPS. At the end of the procedure we had obtained pure extracts of Borrelia LPS with which to test our theory.

We carried out two series of experiments. In the first series we injected both humans and rabbits with pure LPS. The results were striking: rabbits that received the LPS intravenously became feverish within a few hours, and rabbits and humans who received injections of LPS under the skin developed an ECM-like rash.

In our second series of experiments we wanted to observe both the in vivo and the in vitro responses of human macrophages (which synthesize IL-1) to B. burgdorferi. We cultured the two cell types together and found that the macrophages secrete large quantities of IL-1 in the presence of the spiro-

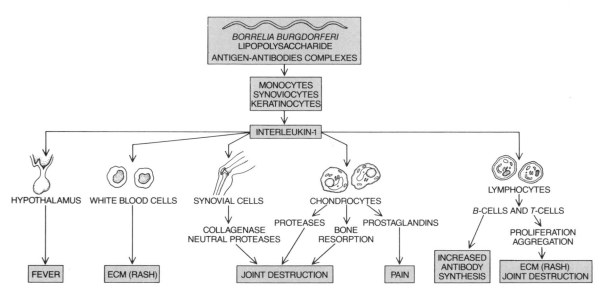

Figure 3.7 LIPOPOLYSACCHARIDES from the spirochete *Borrelia burgdorferi* trigger the release of interleukin-1, which plays a major role in the pathogenesis of Lyme disease. The IL-1 acts on various organs and cells to pro-

duce symptoms such as the rash, fever and arthritis that characterize stages one, two and three of Lyme disease. The spirochete (*top*) is enlarged roughly 1,000 diameters.

chete. Then we examined thin sections of rabbit skin that had been injected intradermally with either IL-1, *B. burgdorferi* or LPS. All were capable of inducing an acute inflammatory response in the skin. We therefore believe that both the skin lesions and the fever can be explained by the release of IL-1.

We also believe that IL-1 released in response to *Borrelia* is directly responsible for the arthritis characterizing the third stage of Lyme disease. When IL-1 is put into culture with cells from the synovium, the inner lining of a human joint such as the knee, it stimulates production of two compounds: the enzyme collagenase and a substance called prostaglandin. Both contribute to arthritis. Collagenase does so by degrading collagen, the primary component of the connective tissue in joints; the degradation leads to a pattern of erosion much like the one seen in severe cases of Lyme arthritis. Prostaglandin contributes to arthritis by promoting pain. Our experiments also show that synovial cells from Lyme disease patients release IL-1 when the cells are exposed to either *Borrelia* or LPS extracts from *Borrelia*.

The Jarisch-Herxheimer reaction experienced by some Lyme disease patients is consistent with our theory: antibiotic treatment kills large numbers of the spirochetes at the same time, releasing large quantities of LPS into the bloodstream and triggering the production of IL-1.

Much remains to be learned about Lyme disease. Currently there are no effective control programs; the best protection against it is caution in tick-infested areas and sensitivity to the early warning signs of the disease. Although our research on the role of IL-1 may not contribute to the control of the disease, we believe our work may have significance beyond this single illness. By examining the physiological response to infection we have shown how a single infectious agent can set off a chain reaction, and how the localized production of a powerful biological mediator such as IL-1 may account for the inflammatory changes characteristic of Lyme arthritis. We hope this will be a useful model for other arthritic diseases of unknown origin.

POSTSCRIPT

The naming of diseases is an interesting matter. Legionellosis received its name in recognition of the fact that it was first discovered in a group of individuals attending an American Legion convention in Philadelphia. Bubonic plague was so named because the swollen lymph nodes of the groin or armpits that are a common symptom were called bubos, from the Latin *bubon*, meaning, literally, groin. Lyme disease acquired its name from the town of Lyme, Connecticut, where it was first recognized as a disease entity. Although the people of Lyme may not enjoy the notoriety they have achieved, the name is now fixed in the literature and will most likely not be changed.

The story of Lyme disease is another story in medical detective work. Although not as dramatic as the story of legionellosis, it is no less significant. The key to Lyme disease was the discovery of the role of an arthropod, the deer tick *Ixodes dammini*, in the transmittal of the pathogen. The pathogen itself is a bacterium, a member of the important group called the spirochetes. Although many spirochetes are harmless, a number of spirochetes cause important diseases of animals and humans. The genus *Borrelia*, in which the Lyme disease organism is placed, contains some other important pathogens, including *Borrelia recurrentis*, the causal agent of recurrent fever. The most important spirochetal disease is syphilis, a sexually transmitted disease, caused by *Treponema pallidum*. Syphilis and Lyme disease even seem to share common symptoms, including rashes, arthritis, and neurological complications (in the later stages).

Although legionellosis seems to be an affliction primarily of the elderly, Lyme disease is indiscriminate, affecting all ages and both sexes, as well as dogs and other animals. Although children are more often affected than adults, this is apparently because children more often enter wooded areas where the tick is present. Fortunately, Lyme disease can be readily treated with antibiotics, although therapy is more difficult if the disease has progressed to the third stage. The principal difficulty with Lyme disease is its diagnosis, since the disease is so newly known that few physicians have ever seen a case. Diagnosis is more likely to be accurate in those areas where the disease is already endemic, such as the Atlantic Coast and the Mississippi River area, because in those areas physicians are more likely to be alert to the symptoms. The most effective control at present is to exercise caution in tick-infested areas where Lyme disease has already been identified.

PREVENTION IS BETTER THAN CURE

. . .

Introduction to Section II

There are two major approaches to the control of infectious disease: prevention and cure. Curing an infection already in progress is a medical procedure, requiring the availability of an appropriate drug. Before antibiotics, infection with many pathogenic bacteria was often fatal, but today antibiotics have kept the fatality rates quite low. A vast array of highly effective antibiotics are available for curing bacterial diseases. Unfortunately, antibiotics are expensive, and in many of the less developed parts of the world are beyond the reach of the medical profession. Also, antibiotics are ineffective against viruses, and some of the most important diseases of humans are caused by viruses. Thus, the physician must turn to methods that can prevent infection from getting started.

Prevention of an infectious disease can be done in one of two ways: by public health measures or by vaccines. Public-health measures such as sanitary procedures (water purification, sewage treatment) require a sophisticated societal input. Vaccines, on the other hand, can be prepared with relatively little cost or effort. Long before antibiotics were available, vaccines brought under control some of the most serious infectious diseases. Vaccines remain today the appropriate technology in the underdeveloped countries.

The disease smallpox has been of great importance in the development of modern medicine. Because of certain peculiarities in its habit, smallpox was an especially favorable disease for the development of vaccination procedures, and it is not by chance that the first vaccine ever developed was for smallpox. The success of the smallpox vaccine is one of the most stirring stories in medicine: through a concerted application of the vaccine the disease has been eradicated from the earth. Chapter 4, "Immunization against Smallpox before Jenner," and Chapter 5, "The Eradication of Smallpox," tell that story.

However, there are major obstacles to repeating the smallpox story for other diseases. In the underdeveloped countries, the use of vaccines presents major problems, which is especially tragic because in those countries death rates from infectious disease are especially high, and infectious disease falls primarily on young children. However, Chapter 6, "Obstacles to Developing Vaccines for the Third World," puts forth the hope that through the intensive efforts of the World Health Organization, major inroads will be made into infectious disease in the underdeveloped parts of the world.

Finally, Chapter 7, "Synthetic Vaccines," provides some fascinating insights into future developments that biotechnology will bring to the vaccine world. Although synthetic vaccines have not yet been used in medicine, the procedures for development of such vaccines are now available and hold considerable promise for the future.

Immunization against Smallpox before Jenner

Long before he introduced inoculation with cowpox, smallpox was prevented by inoculation with smallpox itself. The procedure was risky, but its spread in the 18th century set the stage for Jenner.

. . .

William L. Langer
January, 1976

In the 17th century smallpox, a disease that is now on the verge of eradication, was endemic everywhere in Europe and probably throughout the world. Perhaps the most infectious disease of humans, it was in many respects even more loathsome and fearful than that other great killer, plague. Where plague decided between life and death within three or four days (see Chapter 1, "The Bubonic Plague", smallpox lasted for two weeks or longer. Its first signs were fever, backache and vomiting. The fever then subsided, and many small bumps the size of birdshot appeared on the skin, particularly on the face, the chest and the arms. Over several days the bumps enlarged as they filled with fluid. The fever then returned and the bumps became inflamed and swollen pustules that broke and formed a soft yellow crust with an offensive odor. Eventually, if the patient survived (and in many epidemics two in five died), the crusts fell off, revealing the characteristic pox or depressed scars, that gave the disease it name (see Figure 4.1). It was not unusual for the patient also to be left blind.

Although smallpox most commonly attacked children under five, it did not respect age or social status. Scarcely 20 percent of the population escaped it entirely, and it was always more virulent in the cities than it was in the countryside. In 17th-century London it accounted for some 10 percent of all deaths, and it took an even higher toll in other European cities. Like plague it would assume epidemic proportions every five to 10 years. About 1660, just as plague was beginning to die out in Europe, the threat from smallpox increased. Not long afterward the intelligentsia of Europe awakened to a fact already known to common folk: this terrifying scourge was avoidable. Smallpox was in fact the first major disease that was amenable to a form of prophylaxis; it could not be cured but it could be prevented.

Today the prevention of smallpox is usually associated with the name of Edward Jenner, but in many parts of the Old World people had practiced one method or another of "buying the pox" long before Jenner's time. Fearful for their children's health, parents would seek out someone with a case of smallpox, preferably a mild one. The smallpox vic-

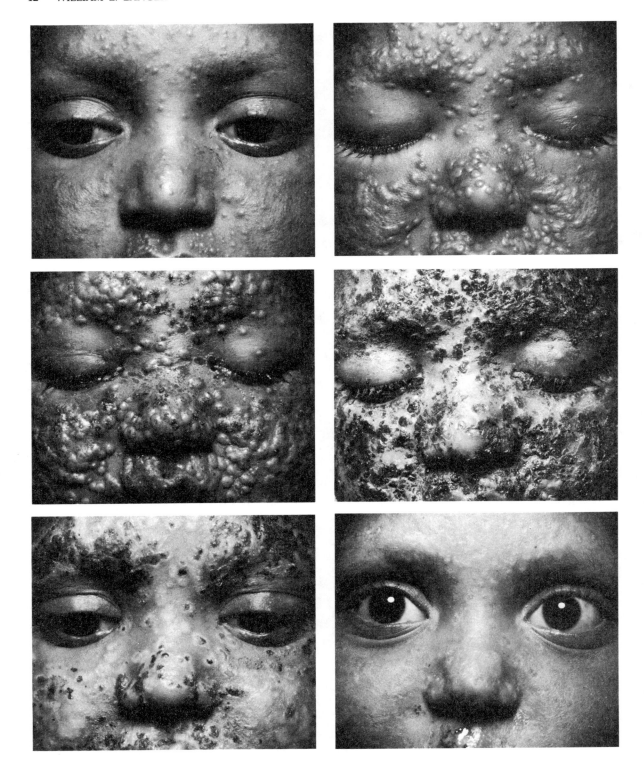

Figure 4.1 DEVELOPMENT OF SMALLPOX in a child is shown in this series of photographs made under the auspices of the World Health Organization. The first photograph (*top left*) was made on the third day after the smallpox rash had first appeared; the remaining photographs (*left to right and top to bottom*) were made on fifth, seventh, 10th, 15th and 25th days. In the course of the infection the rash develops into pustules, which in this case have begun to break on the seventh day. By the 25th day the pustules have largely healed, leaving the depressed scars characteristic of the disease.

tim and the child would then make contact in such a way as to infect the child. After an incubation period of about a week the child, if he was lucky, would develop a mild case of smallpox and would emerge virtually unscarred and immune to the disease thereafter; the mild induced case gave the same protection that was provided by a severe one. Educated people came to call this practice of folk medicine inoculation, after the Latin *inoculare*, to graft. They also called it variolation; variola, from the Latin *varus*, pimple, was the scholarly name for smallpox.

There were numerous techniques of variolation. The Chinese avoided direct contact with the sick; instead the child was induced to inhale a powder made from the crusts shed by a recovering patient. In the Near East and in Africa fresh material from a diseased patient's pustules was rubbed into a cut or scratch in the skin of the person being immunized. The first scholarly account of peasant immunization practices in Europe appears to be one written by Thomas Bartholin, an anatomist at the University of Copenhagen and later physician to Christian V, king of Denmark and Norway; his note on variolation in the Danish countryside was published in 1675. At that time the practice was also known in rural France and in Wales.

In England 40 more years passed before the folk practices came to the notice of the learned. An Oxford-trained Greek physician then living in Constantinople, Emanuel Timoni, was the reporter. He wrote to the Royal Society of London in 1713 to describe to his fellow members the method of variolation used in the Near East. His note (see Figure 4.2) was summarized in the society's *Philosophical Transactions* in 1714. Two years later the same journal published a more detailed analysis of the Eastern practice written by an Italian physician, James Pylarini, who was then serving as the British consul in Smyrna. Variolation was practiced in Smyrna along well-established Near Eastern lines; profes-

sional variolators, usually women, took material from a ripe pustule and rubbed it into a scratch or an incision in the arm or leg of the person being inoculated.

We now come to Mary Pierrepont, a well-born English beauty who against her father's wishes eloped in 1712 with Edward Wortley Montagu, a grandson of the first earl of Sandwich. The couple lived quietly in the country until Edward became a member of Parliament for Westminster in 1715 and his wife suddenly found herself one of the most popular hostesses in London and a friend of the leading intellectuals of the capital. That same year Lady Mary contracted smallpox, to the ruin of her beauty. The following year her husband was sent as ambassador to the Turkish court in Constantinople. Lady Mary, who now had an understandable interest in smallpox, was greatly impressed by what she saw of the Turkish practice of variolation. She had the embassy physician inoculate her young son, and on her return to London in 1718 she agitated enthusiastically in favor of variolation. When her daughter reached the age of four in 1721, Lady Mary made sure that she too was inoculated against smallpox. Although she was not the first to report the Eastern practice to the English, Lady Mary deserves great credit both for her courage in having her children inoculated and for her persistent propaganda in court circles.

Lady Mary and those physicians who, having read the Royal Society reports, also favored the practice met with sustained and not entirely irrational opposition. Many clergymen simply denounced variolation as an interference with God's will. The fact remains that a few of those who were inoculated did die. More important, all who were inoculated became potential sources of contagion throughout the period of their illness.

Curiously, this contagious effect had not been foreseen and might have continued to go unnoticed except for an incident in the country north of London. The physician who had variolated Lady Mary's son in Constantinople had by now returned to England and happened to variolate the daughter of a Hertford Quaker. The household staff was large, and in the course of the little girl's illness and convalescence six of the servants (who had never contracted smallpox and therefore had no immunity) came in close contact with the child. All six were stricken, and a local epidemic ensued. Thus although a certain degree of progress was achieved

V. *An Account, or History, of the Procuring the* SMALL POX *by Incision, or Inoculation; as it has for some time been practised at* Constantinople.

Being the Extract of a Letter from Emanuel Timonius, Oxon. & Patav. M. D. S. R. S. *dated at* Constantinople, December, 1713.

Communicated to the Royal Society *by* John Woodward, M. D. Prof. Med. Gresh. *and* S. R. S.

THE Writer of this ingenious Discourse observes, in the first place, that the *Circassians, Georgians,* and other *Asiaticks,* have introduc'd this Practice of procuring the *Small-Pox* by a sort of Inoculation, for about the space of forty Years, among the *Turks* and others at *Constantinople.*

That altho' at first the more prudent were very cautious in the use of this Practice; yet the happy Success it has been found to have in thousands of Subjects for these eight Years past, has now put it out of all suspicion and doubt; since the Operation having been perform'd on Persons of all

Figure 4.2 FIRST ACCOUNT OF INOCULATION for smallpox to appear in England was written by Emanuel Timoni and published in the *Philosophical Transactions* of the Royal Society of London in 1714. Timoni, then in Constantinople, described the method there.

(George I, for example, allowed the royal grandchildren to be immunized), variolation in England remained the exception rather than the rule.

At the same time inoculation against smallpox was initiated quite independently on the other side of the Atlantic. Boston was then the intellectual center of the British colonies in America, and Cotton Mather, the eminent theologian and far-ranging scholar, was a member of the Royal Society of London. Mather read the society's *Philosophical Transactions,* and soon after the appearance of Timoni's note he wrote a friend in England to say that one of his slaves had already told him of variolation as it was practiced in Africa.

In April, 1721, a smallpox epidemic broke out in Boston. Mather tried to mobilize the physicians of the city for a campaign of immunization. With one exception the response was outspokenly negative. The exception was Zabdiel Boylston. On June 26 Boylston inoculated his six-year-old son, one of his slaves and the slave's three-year-old boy, all with-

out any adverse effects. Boylston thereupon proceeded to inoculate more than 200 other Bostonians in spite of a vigorous newspaper and pamphlet campaign in opposition to the practice (see Figure 4.3). Unlike the opposition in England, Boylston's principal adversaries were his fellow physicians. The clergy on the whole supported Mather and Boylston.

The issue was a grave one, because the 1721 epidemic was unusually severe. Almost half of the population of Boston, 5,889 of the city's 12,000 inhabitants (11,720 if one subtracts the 280 immunized by Boylston and two other physicians), contracted smallpox. Of this number 844, or every seventh victim, died. The next smallpox epidemic to strike Boston, a less severe outbreak in 1730, was met with a much more widespread inoculation program.

Meanwhile in England interest in variolation continued to decline until John Kirkpatrick, an American physician from Charleston, S.C., visited London in 1743. He brought to English medical circles details of how inoculation had successfully halted a

Their Ages.	Persons inoculated.	Had the Small-Pox by Inoculation.	Had an Imperfect small Pox.	Had no Effect.	Suspected to have died of Inoculation.
From 9 months to 2 years old.	06	06	00	00	00
2 to 5	14	14	00	00	00
5 to 10	16	16	00	00	00
10 to 15	29	29	00	00	00
15 to 20	51	51	00	00	01
20 to 30	62	60	00	02	01
30 to 40	44	42	00	02	01
40 to 50	08	07	00	01	00
50 to 60	07	06	00	01	02
60 to 67	07	07	00	00	01
Total	244	238	00	06	06
Inoculated by Drs. Roby and Thompson in Roxbury and Cambridge.	36	36	00	00	00
Total	280	274	00	00	06

Figure 4.3 RECORD OF INOCULATIONS performed in Boston and vicinity by Zabdiel Boylston and two colleagues during the smallpox epidemic of 1721 appears in an account published by Boylston. Those inoculated numbered 280 aged between nine months and 67 years. Six of them died of smallpox. Six others had no reaction; they may already have had the disease.

particularly severe outbreak of smallpox in Charleston in 1738. Kirkpatrick gave credit to an improved method of variation that had reduced the severity of the disease in inoculated patients and had lowered the mortality rate among the immunized to one in 100. (About one in 50 of Boylston's patients had died.)

Kirkpatrick's report reopened the debate over inoculation in England. In 1746 a special facility, the Smallpox and Inoculation Hospital, was founded in London with the patronage of the duke of Marlborough. Although the hospital's capacity was limited, it quickly became a center of study and teaching; many students from abroad went there to learn the techniques of variation. In 1754 Kirkpatrick's account of the success in Charleston was published. Translated into French and other languages, it soon became virtually a catechism. The next year Robert

and Daniel Sutton, father and son, began to practice variation, first in Suffolk and then in London. The Suttons made many improvements in variation technique, and before moving to London they reported that they had inoculated 2,514 individuals without a single fatality. Daniel opened a private clinic in the city and soon attracted an imposing clientele of well-to-do Londoners. It is reported that he earned 2,000 guineas in 1764 and 6,500 the following year.

There is nothing implausible in Sutton's financial success; by the middle of the 18th century, as one authority notes, variation had become a "social institution." Several dozen young physicians, having learned the technique of variation, set up practice on the Continent and made a good living; the situation was much as it is today, when golf clubs on the Continent think that in order to gain prestige they must have a Scottish professional. The clientele, however, continued to be drawn mainly from the upper classes. For example, in 1756 a Geneva physician, Theodore Tronchin, was summoned to Paris to inoculate the family of the Duc d'Orléans, second in rank only to the king. So great was the excitement that elegant carriages formed a queue at Tronchin's door, much as if their owners were attending a performance at the Comédie Française.

In spite of exceptions such as this one, inoculation in Europe remained virtually an English monopoly. When professional inoculators were called in to train a corps of local physicians in the techniques of variolation (for example, a team was called to Potsdam by Frederick the Great and another to Vienna by the Empress Maria Theresa), it was from England that they were summoned. The French did not begin to catch up with the English in this respect until the mid-1750's, after another smallpox epidemic had broken out. With some interruptions the outbreak continued until the 1790's, and during those years the disease attacked a larger percentage of adults than usual.

Voltaire, who had survived an attack of smallpox at the age of 29, was a staunch advocate of inoculation. The prime mover among the French, however, was not Voltaire but a scientist of great eminence, Charles Marie de La Condamine, a mathematician and geographer whose fame sprang from an expedition to the Amazon in the 1730's. La Condamine went into action during the epidemic of the 1750's. In 1754 he published a number of tracts attacking the clergy's will-of-God position (an argument that appears to have been particularly influential in France) and advocated variolation as a means of controlling the epidemic. The Parlement of Paris, the chief judicial body of France, reacted to popular pressure by appointing a commission of 12 from the Faculty of Medicine of the University of Paris to investigate the issue and draft a report.

After much argument the commission split evenly for and against variolation, but when at last it reported the stalemate, the Faculty of Medicine as a whole had already come to favor this means of preventing smallpox. The practice was sanctioned by the Parlement until in 1763 a fresh epidemic in the city (urban areas were always the worst hit) was attributed to the contagion that inevitably accompanied inoculation. The Parlement responded by forbidding variolation within the Paris city limits, but the inoculators reacted to the prohibition by opening clinics just outside the capital. Among those practitioners, in addition to various English professionals and Tronchin, was a Venetian physician, Angelo Gatti, who lived in Paris and contributed substantially to the study of the disease. Five years later the Parlement rescinded its prohibition.

A roster of the better-known victims of the mid-century epidemics dramatizes the fact that smallpox did not respect the rich and powerful. In 1759 the most notable victim was the empress of Austria, Maria Theresa, stricken at the age of 52. She recovered and later engaged a Dutch physician to inoculate the members of the imperial family. In 1774 the most notable victim was the king of France, Louis XV, stricken at 64. After two weeks of agony he died; his malodorous body was hurried to the grave at night for fear that in those troubled times the usual pomp of a royal funeral might provoke a popular uprising. His death so frightened his successor, Louis XVI, that the monarch immediately had the entire royal family inoculated.

Perhaps inspired by Maria Theresa's experience or due to the hideous appearance of her own pock-marked late husband, Czar Peter, Catherine the Great summoned a London physician, Thomas Dimsdale, to St. Petersburg in 1768 to inoculate her and her son and heir, the Grand Duke Paul. This Dimsdale did without mishap in the fall of 1768. The grateful Catherine not only bestowed the title of baron on Dimsdale but also gave him a cash gift of 10,000 pounds (and another 2,000 pounds to cover expenses) and established an annuity of 500 pounds for him: a remarkable compensation to pay anyone for immunity against smallpox. In 1781 Dimsdale made a second journey to Russia to inoculate Catherine's grandsons, Constantine and Alexander. He also immunized many other members of the Russian aristocracy, both in St. Petersburg and in Moscow. Efforts to promote inoculation in Russia at this time were extensive (see Figure 4.4).

By the eve of the French Revolution the method of inoculation had been so improved that a small pinprick and a drop of thin pus inserted by lancet served the purpose. It would probably be safe to say that everywhere in Europe a majority of the well-to-do had been variolated; after all, it was an excellent investment for those who could afford it. Some students of 18th-century population growth have suggested that the widespread practice had noticeably reduced the overall mortality rate in Europe and

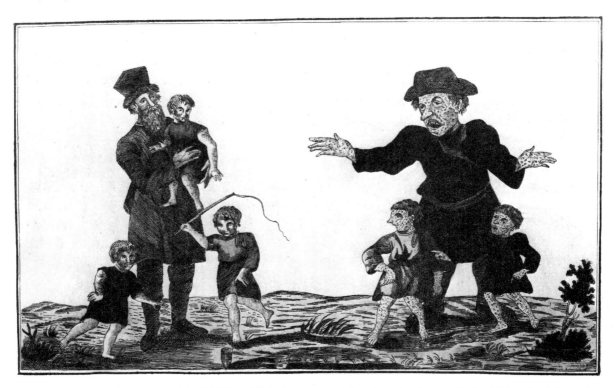

Figure 4.4 PRO-INOCULATION CARTOON published in 18th-century Russia shows a father and children (*left*) whose clear skin contrasts with the disfiguring smallpox scars of another family (*right*). The pockmarked father complains that the "pretty little children" of the other family refuse to play with his "monsters." His disfigured children scold their father for failing to inoculate them.

was thus responsible, at least in part, for the phenomenal increase in population at that time. There can be no certain judgment on the point; it is impossible, first, to establish the death rate for a time before the initiation of the census and, second, to speak with any assurance of the extent of successful immunization. The suggestion does, however, raise a further question: To what extent was variolation practiced among urban and rural workers? The urban poor in particular were the traditional incubators of endemic disease, and they made up the vast majority of the population in all cities. If they were not inoculated, there could be no hope of eradicating smallpox.

The well-to-do were not blind to the problem. Public clinics were opened and in some instances offered free inoculation for children. In England, Jonas Hanway, a well-known philanthropist and a trustee of the Foundling Hospital, suggested to his peers that they employ no servants who had not had smallpox or been inoculated against it. The younger Sutton, whose clinic was perhaps the most elegant in London, offered to variolate 400 children, 100 at a time, and care for them for a full month afterward if rich patrons would subscribe a guinea per head. Nothing came of his proposition, presumably for lack of subscribers.

As for the urban poor themselves, they seem to have shown no great interest in the issue. Naturally suspicious of approaches by their social superiors, they may also have held the pessimistic view that smallpox was an integral part of life. Perhaps they had no reason to think otherwise. Those of them who favored variolation would have looked to itinerant inoculators or even to amateurs for treatment. Such practitioners could not have been relied on to do an up-to-date job. More important, it would have been impossible in the urban slums to isolate the newly inoculated. Inoculated children would not have felt the effects for a week or so and would have continued to be in contact with others. It is reasonable to suppose they would thus have infected other children, who would then have come down with a full-blown case of the disease. If new contagion of this kind was commonplace, it is not hard to understand why many believed smallpox was constantly gaining ground. Contemporary writings contain eloquent testimony to a veritable panic over the disease that seized all Europe in the last quarter of the 18th century.

Much later, in 1852, Thackeray, recalling his life early in the 19th century, noted that at that time hundreds died or rose from their sickbed terribly scarred and disfigured. "In my early days," he wrote in *Henry Esmond*, "this pestilence would enter a village and destroy half the inhabitants: at its approach, it may well be imagined, not only the beautiful but the strongest were alarmed and those fled who could." There is more than enough contemporary evidence to show that Thackeray's remarks were not exaggerated.

Under the circumstances many physicians sought ways to prevent the infection that resulted from variolation. Jenner, a physician with a preference for a country practice, noted in the 1790's that the dairymaids in his neighborhood rarely, if ever, contracted smallpox, even in the absence of inoculation. After years of careful observation and experiment he published in 1798 a 70-page pamphlet: "An Inquiry into the Causes and Effects of the Variolae Vaccinae." (Variolae vaccinae was cowpox, the bovine form of smallpox.) In this classic report (see Figure 4.5) Jenner advanced the notion that inoculation with cowpox, which he considered a mild form of smallpox, would provide the same immunity to smallpox that variolation did. What was more important, the disease produced by vaccination, as opposed to variolation, would be so extremely mild that the vaccinated individual would not be a source of infection.

No better news could have reached the world in the midst of the Napoleonic Wars. Jenner's thesis was accepted at once by the great majority of physicians, and within a year or two thousands had been vaccinated. The news raced around the world faster than news had ever traveled before; Jenner was hailed everywhere as mankind's greatest benefactor, and his discovery was characterized as the most important medical advance of all time.

It is not my purpose here even to touch on the history of vaccination in the 19th and 20th centuries except to note that for all its benefits the procedure was not quite as simple and the immunity it conferred was not as long-lived as Jenner and the early vaccinators had supposed. Nonetheless, it seems appropriate to close this review of the antecedents of Jenner's great discovery with a note on its instant adoption in the U.S.

At the close of the 18th century a highly imaginative (although somewhat eccentric and testy) Harvard professor of medicine, Benjamin Waterhouse, played a role not unlike the one played by Mather and Boylston in the opening decades of the century. Waterhouse had been educated in Europe and maintained a regular correspondence with his friends there. Having received a copy of Jenner's pamphlet almost as soon as it could arrive by ship, Waterhouse was at once converted to Jenner's view. He wrote to friends in England asking for some of the cowpox material used for vaccination. It arrived in July, 1800, and he immediately vaccinated his children and servants.

Waterhouse promptly notified Thomas Jefferson, who was then vice-president, of Jenner's discovery. That always inquisitive statesman at once sought Waterhouse's good offices in securing an ample supply of the vaccine. Jefferson and his son thereupon vaccinated their entire household of 60, slaves included. As president, Jefferson went on to use his influence to establish the new procedure in Philadelphia and the other cities of the young republic. Before Jefferson's retirement to Monticello in 1809 the number of people who had been vaccinated on both sides of the Atlantic could be reckoned in the millions. The campaign to eradicate smallpox, which came to a close in the 1970's (see Chapter 5, "The Eradication of Smallpox"), had begun in earnest.

POSTSCRIPT

In contrast to plague, smallpox is so obviously an infectious disease that its mode of transmission was understood even before the germ theory of disease had been proved. Although most people did not die from smallpox, the disease caused disfiguring lesions on the skin that remained throughout life. No respecter of age or social status, smallpox spread through the nobility as it did through the peasants, and it was therefore understandable that rulers of

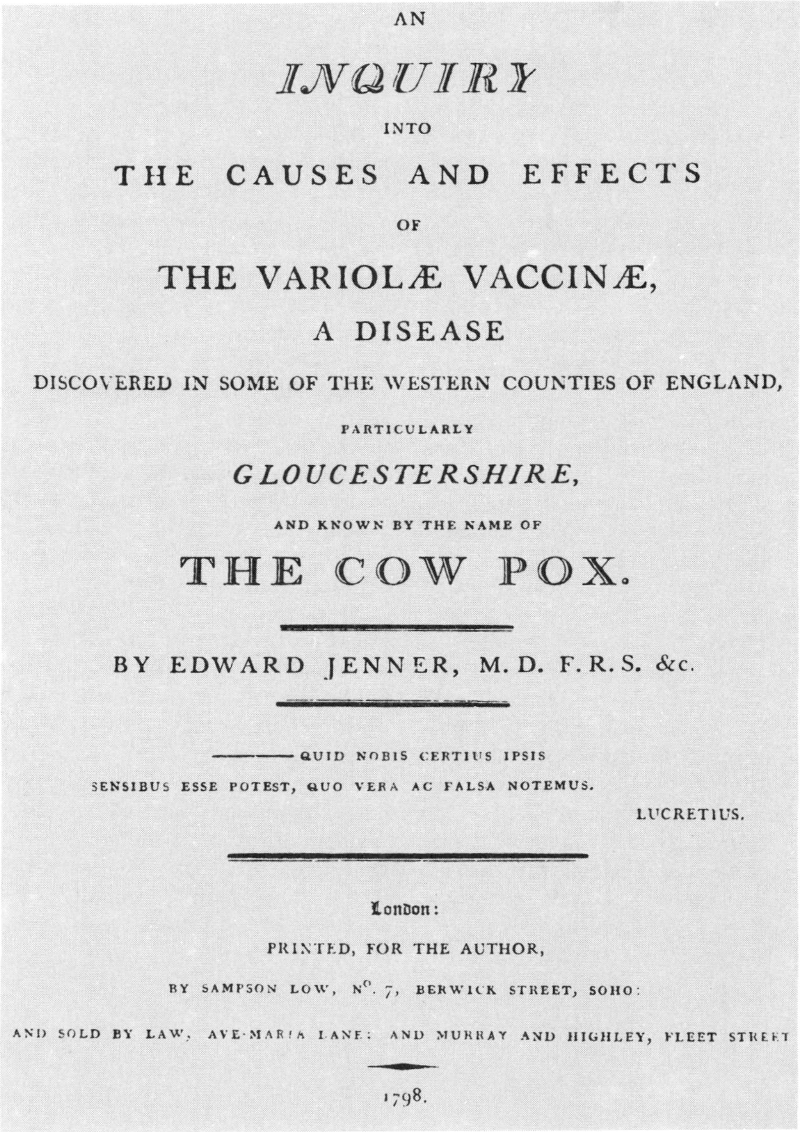

AN

INQUIRY

INTO

THE CAUSES AND EFFECTS

OF

THE VARIOLÆ VACCINÆ,

A DISEASE

DISCOVERED IN SOME OF THE WESTERN COUNTIES OF ENGLAND,

PARTICULARLY

GLOUCESTERSHIRE,

AND KNOWN BY THE NAME OF

THE COW POX.

BY EDWARD JENNER, M.D. F.R.S. &c.

———— QUID NOBIS CERTIUS IPSIS
SENSIBUS ESSE POTEST, QUO VERA AC FALSA NOTEMUS.

LUCRETIUS.

London:

PRINTED, FOR THE AUTHOR,

BY SAMPSON LOW, N°. 7, BERWICK STREET, SOHO:

AND SOLD BY LAW, AVE-MARIA LANE; AND MURRAY AND HIGHLEY, FLEET STREET

1798.

Figure 4.5 INOCULATION WITHOUT CONTAGION, using cowpox pustules instead of smallpox pustules as the source of inoculation material, was proposed by Edward Jenner in 1798. The title page of his pamphlet on the subject is shown here. The quotation is from *De rerum natura,* by Lucretius, a Roman poet of the first century B.C., who suggests that in distinguishing between truth and falsehood man has no more certain criterion than his senses.

the civilized countries would welcome a means of prevention.

In contrast to the diseases discussed in Section I, smallpox is caused not by a bacterium but by a virus. Viruses are infectious agents at the borderline of life and have properties quite different from those of the other disease-causing agents: bacteria, fungi and protozoa. We understand today that a virus is an entity whose properties are determined by its nucleic acid component. By many definitions, viruses are not even living, since they are unable to multiply outside of living tissue; they are thus called obligate parasites. This property, and their submicroscopic size, have made viruses difficult to study, and it was only many years after Koch's postulates had led to the isolation of most of the important bacterial pathogens that viruses came under appropriate laboratory study. However, despite the technical difficulties of studying smallpox, it was the first infectious disease to come under medical control. This was because of the relative ease with which a mild case of smallpox could be introduced into an individual by inoculation. Although Jenner's discovery of the cowpox vaccine was the single most important advance in medicine during the 19th century, the principle of inoculation, using smallpox virus itself, had already been well established before Jenner.

Some of our technical terms come from smallpox. The medical term inoculate was used first for smallpox. The words vaccinate and vaccine, which are in wide use in immunology today, come from Jenner's discovery that cowpox was a mild form of smallpox, and *vacca* is the Latin word for cow.

After Jenner, there was a long hiatus before the next vaccine was developed, by Louis Pasteur in the late 1870's, but Pasteur's work was soon to dramatize the possibilities of preventive medicine. Pasteur developed an inoculation procedure for anthrax, an important bacterial disease of farm animals that also affected humans. Pasteur's procedure involved culturing the anthrax bacillus in such a way that its virulence was weakened but its ability to immunize was not. Pasteur called such a weakened culture attenuated. Recognizing that a weakened anthrax bacillus was analogous to Jenner's cowpox, Pasteur honored Jenner by calling his anthrax inoculation procedure a vaccination, and soon the term was applied to any inoculation procedure using a weakened inoculating agent.

After his success with anthrax, Pasteur turned to rabies, a virus disease transmitted to a human by the bite of an infected animal. Because rabies infection was almost 100 percent fatal, the disease was one of the most feared of human ailments, even though its incidence was low. Because the rabies virus is an obligate parasite, Pasteur used the rabbit as an experimental animal. After painstaking and intense work over many years, Pasteur succeeded in attenuating the rabies virus and developing a successful vaccine. Because the onset of rabies is slow, it was possible to vaccinate even after infection had occurred. Whereas the smallpox vaccine was a prevention against future attack, the rabies vaccine could actually interfere with an infection already in progress. Soon, people who had been bitten by rabid animals were flocking to Pasteur's laboratory in Paris for the "Pasteur treatment." Public subscription brought in enough money so that a Pasteur Institute was set up in Paris, not only as a center for the Pasteur treatment, but for research on all infectious diseases. By the end of the 19th century, the idea of vaccination had become widely accepted and several other serious infectious diseases of humans had come under control. But no disease has more completely succumbed to vaccination than smallpox. As we will see in Chapter 5, "The Eradication of Smallpox," vaccination has succeeded in eradicating smallpox from the face of the earth.

The Eradication of Smallpox

A 10-year campaign led by the World Health Organization is right now at the point of success. The world may have seen its last case of the most devastating disease in human history.

. . .

Donald A. Henderson
October, 1976

Smallpox, the most devastating and feared pestilence in human history, is making its last stand in two remote areas of Ethiopia, one in the desert and one in the mountains. As of the end of August, 1976, only five villages had experienced cases in the preceding eight weeks. More important, the onset of the last known case was on August 9. Because humans are the only known reservoir for the smallpox virus, the disease should be eliminated forever when the last infected person recovers. Right now more than 1,000 Ethiopian health workers, together with 10 epidemiologists of the World Health Organization, are combing the countryside to make sure no more cases exist (see Figure 5.1). If they discover one, the victim will be isolated under 24-hour guard and everyone who has been in contact with him will be vaccinated. An effort will be made to trace the chain of infection back to a previously known contained outbreak. For two years after the last case is recorded the search will continue for additional outbreaks. If none is found, and if a WHO international commission can be satisfied that the search has been thorough, smallpox will be declared to have been eradicated from the earth. It will be the first such achievement in medical history.

The interruption of smallpox transmission in 1976 was the objective of a 10-year global campaign voted by the World Health Assembly (the WHO's controlling body) in 1966 and launched in 1967. When the campaign began, smallpox was considered to be endemic—an indigenous, ever present illness—in more than 30 countries, and "imported" cases were regularly reported every year in perhaps a dozen other countries. The program moved forward steadily, with major campaigns eliminating smallpox successively in western and central Africa, Brazil, Indonesia, southern Africa, Pakistan, India and Bangladesh (see Figure 5.2). In Ethiopia, the last infected country, the campaign has been complicated by some of the most rugged and inaccessible terrain in Africa; it is estimated that more than half of the country's 28 million people live more than a day's walk from any road. Fighting between government forces and various dissident groups has been a recurrent problem. Two Ethiopian health workers have been shot and killed, and the search teams have had to withdraw from some districts for

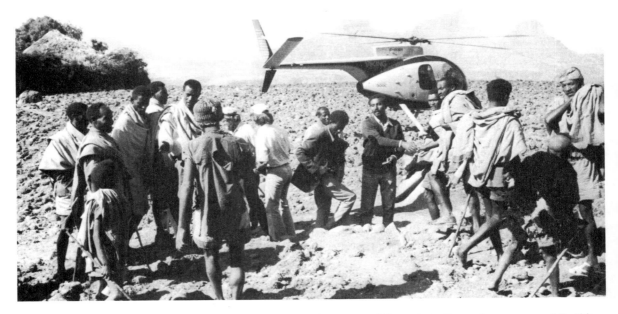

Figure 5.1 SEARCH FOR SMALLPOX CASES is pressed in the remote Simyen Mountains of Ethiopia's Begemdir Province. Two-person teams are assigned to cover an area on foot or on muleback, looking for new cases and vaccinating any possible contacts. Supervisory personnel (in this case a World Health Organization epidemiologist and an Ethiopian counterpart) maintain contact with the teams by helicopter.

weeks at a time. Yet ever since 1971, when the Ethiopian campaign began, both the extent of the infected areas and the number of cases have been steadily reduced (see Figure 5.3), and now final success seems to be within reach.

Smallpox is caused by a virus that spreads from person to person in minute droplets discharged from the mouth or the nose. (Virus particles in clothing or bedding have sometimes infected people who have not had face-to-face contact with a patient, but such indirect infection has been infrequent.) About 10 or 12 days after inhaling the virus the infected person becomes sick, with a high fever and aching sensations resembling those of acute influenza. After two to four days a rash develops on the face, and within a day or two it spreads over the entire body (see Figure 5.4). Usually it has a "centrifugal" distribution: it is densest on the face, arms and legs and less dense on the trunk. The small, red, pimplelike papules quickly become enlarged vesi-

cles filled first with a clear serum and then, by the fifth day of the rash, with pus. In severe cases the pustules may be so close together, particularly on the face and eyelids, that there is no normal skin; the face is swollen and the patient, now acutely ill, may be unrecognizable. By the 10th day scabs begin to form, and by the third week they fall off, leaving depigmented areas that become pitted, disfiguring scars. Some patients are left blind. Among those afflicted by the virulent Asian form of the virus, variola major, from 20 to 40 percent die. In Ethiopia, where the less virulent variola minor is prevalent, the death rate is 1 percent. Once smallpox has been contracted there is no effective treatment for it.

The origin of smallpox antedates written history. The mummified head of the Egyptian pharaoh Ramses V, who died about 1160 B.C. of an acute infection, shows lesions that appear to be those of smallpox. Chinese and Sanskrit texts indicate that smallpox was also present at least that early in China and India. On the other hand, there is no

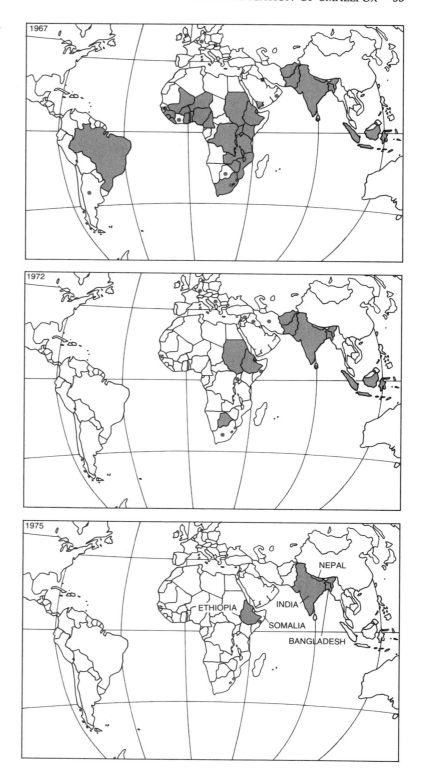

Figure 5.2 GLOBAL CONTRACTION OF SMALLPOX as shown on maps for 1967 (*top*), 1972 (*middle*) and 1975 (*bottom*). The countries where the disease was considered endemic, or indigenous, are shaded in color; those reporting imported cases are designated by a colored dot.

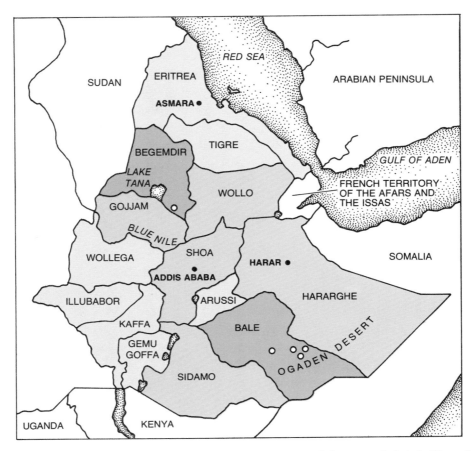

Figure 5.3 IN ETHIOPIA all 14 provinces were infected with smallpox in 1971, when the WHO-directed eradication program began. At the end of 1974 seven provinces (*medium and dark color*) still remained infected. At the end of August 1976 there were infected villages (*white dots*) in only two provinces (*dark color*), in the gorge of the Blue Nile and in the Ogaden Desert.

mention of a disease resembling smallpox in either the Old Testament or the New or in Greek or Roman literature, and it would seem that such a serious disease would almost certainly have been described if it had been prevalent.

A plausible explanation lies in the same epidemiological characteristics of smallpox that lead us to believe it can now be eliminated. Since there is no known animal or insect reservoir of the virus, for infection to persist in a population one afflicted person must transmit the virus to a susceptible contact, and that contact in turn must transmit it to another in an unbroken chain. The smallpox victim can transmit the disease only from the time his rash appears until the scabs drop off, a period of about four weeks. After that he is immune to reinfection. In isolated villages and among scattered populations a point is therefore reached where so few people remain susceptible that the chain of transmission is broken. In such an area smallpox dies out, and it does not recur unless it is reintroduced.

It seems reasonable to speculate that in ancient times only the more densely populated areas of India and China were able to sustain the continued transmission of smallpox. If it was occasionally introduced into less populated central and western Asia, Europe and Africa, it might have persisted for a time in such a region as the Nile delta, but eventually the chain of transmission would have been broken. The slow pace of travel in pre-Christian times

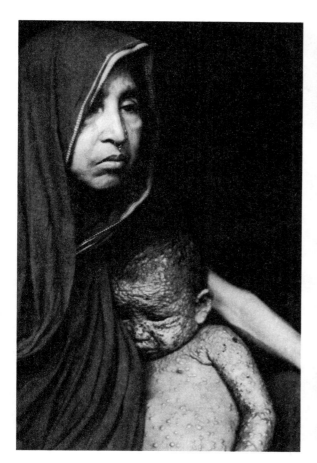

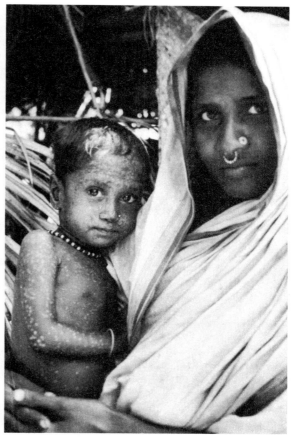

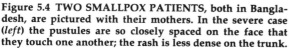

Figure 5.4 TWO SMALLPOX PATIENTS, both in Bangladesh, are pictured with their mothers. In the severe case (*left*) the pustules are so closely spaced on the face that they touch one another; the rash is less dense on the trunk.

The three-year-old girl recovering from smallpox (*right*) was the last known victim in Bangladesh and thus the world's last known case of the more virulent form of the disease, variola major.

and the infrequency of long journeys could have served to confine smallpox largely to Asia during that period. In the early Christian Era, however, descriptions of a disease that was almost certainly smallpox appear increasingly in historical accounts of western Asia and, beginning in the sixth century, of Europe and Africa. In 1520 Spanish conquistadors brought the disease to the Americas.

Increasing population densities provided enough susceptible individuals to sustain the chain of transmission. So pervasive was the disease that, like chickenpox in our time, virtually everyone contracted it. English parish records of the early 18th century indicate that about 20 percent of all small-

pox victims died but that the rate was higher in many epidemics. In one well-documented instance in Iceland in 1707, 18,000 people, or 31 percent of a population of 57,000 died of smallpox. Since part of the population was immune because of previous smallpox, the death rate in that epidemic may have approached 50 percent. (See Chapter 11, "Island Epidemics," on the value of Iceland as a natural laboratory for the study of epidemics.) In Mexico 3.5 million indigenous people are believed to have died of smallpox shortly after it was introduced in the 16th century. Until the advent of vaccination smallpox played a major role in inhibiting population growth.

Even before Edward Jenner's day some people had been protected against smallpox by variolation: material from the pustules of a patient was scratched into the skin of a healthy person, who, if all went well, developed a mild case and was subsequently immune (see Chapter 4, "Immunization against Smallpox before Jenner"). Variolation spread from Asia via the Near East into Europe as a folk practice, and in the early 18th century it was taken up and popularized by physicians in England. The death rate from variolation was only about a tenth as high as the mortality from the naturally acquired disease, but a variolated person could transmit virulent smallpox to others. When variolation became widespread in England, it was common knowledge that dairymaids who had contracted the illness called cowpox would not "take the smallpox" when they were variolated and also appeared to be immune to natural smallpox infection. In 1796 Jenner inoculated material from a dairymaid's cowpox lesion into the arm of an eight-year-old boy, who was subsequently immune to the effects of smallpox variolation. Jenner called the new procedure vaccination, and he predicted that "the annihilation of smallpox must be the final result of this practice." The new technique spread rapidly, but it is only now, as the result of a concerted international public-health effort, that Jenner's prediction is being fulfilled.

Until late in the 19th century virus for vaccination was obtained from the pustular lesion of one vaccinated person and was scratched into the arm of other individuals to be vaccinated. It was an inefficient system, and not infrequently the syphilis spirochete and hepatitis virus were transferred along with the vaccine virus. The discovery that large amounts of vaccine virus could be obtained by scarifying and inoculating the shaved flank of a calf was an important advance. (That procedure is still followed to obtain sufficient quantities of virus for vaccine production.) Preservation of the virus was difficult, however, particularly in tropical climates. Sometimes the calf was led from door to door and a bit of pus was scraped from its flank for each vaccination, but usually the pustular material scraped from the calf was suspended in a 50 percent solution of glycerol in order to reduce bacterial contamination and was distributed in small glass capillaries. In this form and without refrigeration the vaccine remained potent for perhaps a few days.

Jenner himself had noted that dried vaccine lasted longer than liquid vaccine, but for years there was no way to produce dried vaccine in bulk. Methods for the commercial freeze-drying of biological preparations were developed just before World War II, and in the early 1950's a technique for producing a remarkably heat-stable freeze-dried smallpox vaccine was devised by Leslie H. Collier of the Lister Institute in England. Instead of drying the crude pulp scraped from the animal, Collier produced a partly purified suspension of virus by differential centrifugation and freeze-dried the material in the ampules in which it was to be distributed. It was reconstituted with a glycerol solution for the vaccination. Most batches of Collier's vaccine were still potent after storage for two years at body temperature. Potent dried vaccine was an essential tool that could make the eradication of smallpox possible.

In 1926, when the Health Section of the League of Nations began publishing a weekly bulletin on disease prevalence around the world, smallpox was made a reportable disease, but only against opposition. When a Japanese delegate to the International Sanitary Conference suggested that smallpox be made reportable, a Swiss delegate maintained that "smallpox has, in reality, no place in an international convention. It is not a pestilential disease in the proper sense of the term: it is, in effect, a disease that exists everywhere. There is probably not a single country of which it can be said that there are no cases of smallpox."

When the WHO was established in 1948 as a specialized agency of the United Nations, it approached the smallpox problem gingerly at first; its interim commission had stated in 1946 that it was "impracticable as yet" even to standardize smallpox vaccines. By the late 1940's, however, the concept of disease eradication in general and the idea of eradicating smallpox in particular was acquiring a growing number of supporters, one of the most persuasive being Fred L. Soper, director of what was then the Pan American Sanitary Bureau and is now the WHO Regional Office for the Americas. They pointed to the very practical demonstration of the elimination of smallpox from North America and Europe in the 1940's and also—a more notable achievement—from a few countries with less highly developed health services, such as the Philippines and some countries in Central America. A campaign to eradicate smallpox in the Americas was undertaken in 1950, with the Pan American Sanitary Bureau providing technical assistance. The results were encouraging: by 1959 smallpox had been effectively eliminated from all American countries except Argentina, Brazil, Colombia, Ecuador and Bolivia.

In that year, on the initiative of the U.S.S.R., the World Health Assembly called for global smallpox eradication and vaccination "in foci where the disease exists." The resolution pointed out that "funds devoted to the control of and vaccination against smallpox throughout the world exceed those necessary for the eradication of smallpox in its endemic foci."

The WHO and the UN Children's Fund (UNICEF) helped a number of countries to establish vaccine-production centers. Donations of vaccine were received from several countries, and mass-vaccination programs were started by some. Progress was slow, however. A global program to wipe out malaria (see Chapter 8, "The Biochemistry of Resistance to Malaria") had captured the interest and energies of some governments and health workers, and when it faltered, many came to doubt the feasibility of any disease-eradication program. Lack of skilled personnel, vehicles and other necessary assistance kept many countries from undertaking campaigns. Those that did make the attempt were often beset by cases of smallpox imported from adjacent countries. Vaccine donations were far too small to meet the need, and there was no mechanism for regular monitoring of the quality of vaccine produced in newly established production centers. Vaccine quality declined, and countries that found themselves administering poor vaccines became disillusioned.

In 1966 delegates to the World Health Assembly argued that either enough money should be provided for a fully coordinated program or the idea of global smallpox eradication should be given up. After lengthy debate and in spite of many misgivings the delegates voted a special budget of $2.5 million for an intensive program to begin on January 1, 1967. The objective was to eliminate smallpox from the world by the end of 1976.

In 1967, the year the intensified eradication program began, smallpox was considered to be endemic in 33 countries, and 11 others reported cases

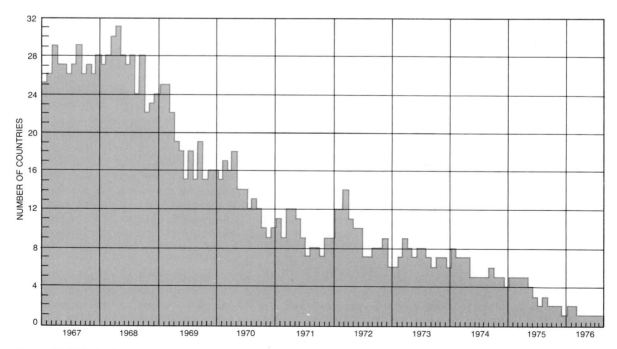

Figure 5.5 TEN-YEAR TREND in the incidence of smallpox is traced here by a histogram showing the number of countries reporting one case or more each month. That includes cases in countries where the disease was endemic and also cases "imported" into nonendemic countries.

attributable to importations (see Figure 5.5). In the Americas, Brazil was the only endemic country, but it alone constituted half a continent. In the rest of the world there were three major reservoirs of smallpox. One, in Asia, extended from what is now Bangladesh through India, Nepal and Pakistan into Afghanistan. A second reservoir comprised virtually all of Africa south of the Sahara. The third reservoir was the Indonesian archipelago.

At the start of the program the urgent need was for adequate supplies of potent and stable freeze-dried vaccine. Little satisfactory freeze-dried vaccine was being produced anywhere. Some vaccines lacked potency when they were reconstituted and others quickly lost their potency under field conditions; some that were being administered contained no detectable virus whatever. Almost no vaccine in the endemic countries met the WHO's basic standards, and there was no central laboratory for testing vaccines.

At the WHO's request two major laboratories agreed early in the campaign to serve as international vaccine reference centers: the Rijksinstituut voor de Volksgezondheid in the Netherlands and Connaught Laboratories, Ltd., of Toronto. It was estimated that 250 million doses of vaccine a year would be needed for the endemic areas. Buying that amount would have cost more money than had been set aside for the entire program, and so a decision was made not to buy any vaccine but to ask for donations of it, and to provide equipment and technical advice to laboratories within the endemic regions so that at least the most populous endemic countries could produce good vaccine on their own.

In the first years most of the vaccine — more than 140 million doses a year — was given by the U.S.S.R. and 40 million doses came from the U.S. Eventually donations were received from more than 20 countries. Gradually vaccine production in the developing countries increased and the quality improved, until by 1970 all the vaccine in the program met accepted international standards of potency and stability.

Another early objective was to simplify and improve the vaccination techniques. The commonest technique throughout the world when the program began was some form of the scratch method: a drop of vaccine was placed on the skin and scratched into the superficial layers, sometimes with instruments that made severe wounds. The technique was wasteful of vaccine and achieved a lower success rate than an alternative method in which a needle is held parallel to the skin and the tip is pressed into the skin repeatedly. This multiple-pressure procedure is difficult to follow and to teach, however. A more efficient method that consumed less vaccine was needed.

A jet injector, originally designed for a deeper, subcutaneous injection but modified to accomplish the more superficial smallpox vaccination, had been developed by the U.S. Army. Under high pressure it injected a tenth of a milliliter of vaccine into the superficial layers of the skin. The gun required a more highly purified vaccine than the scratch methods but less than a third as much virus, and more than 1,000 people an hour could be vaccinated with the gun (if that many could be gathered together). Introduced in 1967 for programs in Brazil and Zaire and in 20 countries of western and central Africa assisted by the U.S. Centers for Disease Control, the jet guns proved to be effective, but they were expensive and required considerable maintenance and repair, making them impractical in places where trained technicians were unavailable. And they were of limited benefit in Asia, where vaccination traditionally was done on a house-to-house basis.

The ultimate solution, the bifurcated needle, was developed at Wyeth Laboratories in the 1960's (see Figure 5.6). It resembles a large, blunt sewing needle with part of the eye ground off to leave two small prongs. The bifurcated end of the needle is dipped into the vaccine, and one drop, enough for one vaccination, clings between the prongs. The needle is held perpendicular to the skin and 15 quick punctures are made. Only one-fourth as much vaccine is required as for the scratch technique. Wyeth waived patent charges for the design for any manufacturer producing the needles exclusively for the WHO program. The needle had originally been designed to be used once, but the WHO had them made of special steel so that they could be boiled or flamed more than 200 times without becoming dull.

Vaccination technique was further simplified after field studies revealed that there was no difference in the incidence of bacterial infections whether or not the vaccination site had first been swabbed with acetone, alcohol or soap. That made it possible to dispense with cotton swabs and bottles of soap and alcohol. The vaccinator needs only a vial of

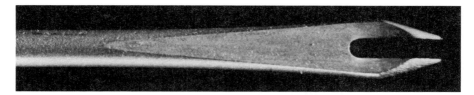

Figure 5.6 BIFURCATED NEEDLE was the principal tool of the vaccination program. The simple instrument was developed by Wyeth Laboratories. The pronged end of the needle is enlarged about 10 diameters in this photograph; the actual length of the needle is about two inches.

diluent for the vaccine, a container of sterile needles and another container for used needles, all of which fit handily into a shirt pocket.

At the beginning of the program there were heavily endemic areas, but it was not at all clear how prevalent the disease was, or how extensive. It quickly became apparent that routine reporting of smallpox cases, particularly in the endemic parts of the world, was far worse than had been supposed; it was so bad that for certain years some large areas were reported as having more smallpox deaths than they had cases. One study in northern Nigeria indicated that the efficiency of reporting was 8.1 percent in an urban area and 1.3 percent in rural areas; in West Java it appeared that not more than 6 percent of all cases had been reported. In the light of nine years of experience we now believe that when the program began not more than 1 percent of all cases were actually being reported. Although 131,418 cases of smallpox worldwide were reported to the WHO in 1967, there may have been that many cases in northern Nigeria alone. An accurate figure for the world in 1967 might be on the order of 10 to 15 million cases.

A major problem was that even when cases were detected and reported by health units they were not necessarily included in national reports. At the time the campaign began in Indonesia only about half of the cases reported at the provincial level were being reported nationally; in Niger, of 325 cases reported to local government units between December, 1966, and February, 1967, only 14 were finally reported to the ministry of health. A first step in national smallpox-eradication campaigns was therefore to increase the quality and regularity of reporting from all fixed medical units. One approach was to appoint a surveillance team of two to four people for each administrative division with two to five million in population. These teams circulated among the medical units encouraging them to report, looking for cases, distributing vaccine, counseling and cajoling.

When the intensified eradication program began, the basic strategy called for a two- to three-year mass-vaccination campaign throughout a country, during which an improved reporting and surveillance system would be developed. It was felt that if 80 percent of the population could be vaccinated, smallpox incidence would be reduced to fewer than five cases per 100,000 of population; thereafter, with improved surveillance, the remaining foci would be identified quickly and measures could be taken to eliminate them.

A development early in the campaign resulted in a change in that strategy. There was a delay in the delivery of supplies for the mass-vaccination program in eastern Nigeria, and an energetic U.S. adviser, William H. Foege, organized an interim program: he searched out smallpox cases and vaccinated thoroughly in a limited area surrounding each case (see Figure 5.7). The mass-campaign supplies arrived only a few months later, but by then there was no detectable smallpox in eastern Nigeria. And less than half of the population had ever been vaccinated.

This result and similar experiences in other places led to an emphasis, even in the early stage of the campaigns, on what became known as surveillance-containment: improved search and detection as speedily as possible, isolation of patients and vaccination of every known or suspected contact around them. The procedure sealed off outbreaks from the rest of the population. That proved to be effective partly because in most areas smallpox turned out to spread slower than had been supposed. One person

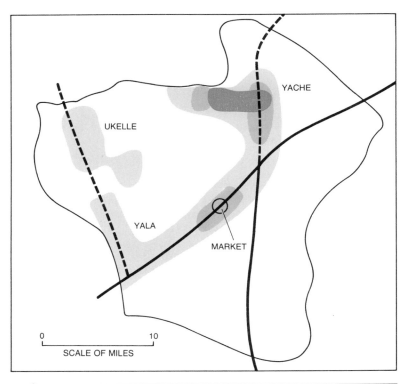

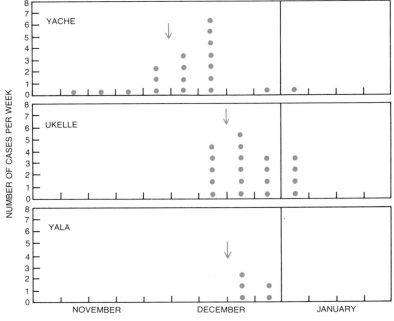

Figure 5.7 OUTBREAK IN NI-
GERIA at the outset of the campaign was dealt with by containment. The outbreak was reported
on December 4, 1966, in Yache, a
village in the Ogojn district (*map
at top*). Vaccination began that
day in the area (*dark color*) immediately surrounding the known
cases and was extended, as new
cases were reported, to successively implicated areas (*medium
color and light color*). The table
(*bottom*) relates cases by week of
onset to the initiation of vaccination. In each village the outbreak
was ended within two or three
weeks after vaccination began
(*arrows*), except for two individuals in Yache who were not successfully immunized.

generally infected no more than two to five others; cases were usually clustered in one part of a town or in adjacent villages rather than being widely and evenly distributed through a country. The containment teams could focus on problem areas and had somewhat more time than had been anticipated in which to seal off an outbreak. When it became clear that smallpox in a previously vaccinated person was uncommon even if the vaccination had been done many years before, heavy emphasis was placed on primary vaccination. (In Asia 80 percent of all cases were reported among the 20 percent of the people who had no vaccination scar.)

Substantial progress was made in the four years after 1967. In 1971 only 16 countries reported smallpox cases. In the 20 countries of western and central Africa where the U.S. Centers for Disease Control was providing support the last case was recorded (in Nigeria) in June, 1970, a full year earlier than had been expected. Elsewhere in Africa endemic smallpox was limited to Ethiopia, whose program did not begin until 1971, to the southern Sudan, where civil war had made a program impossible, and to Botswana, which had been reinfected at about the time of the last cases in neighboring South Africa. Brazil's last case developed in April, 1971, and Indonesia's in January, 1972. One major reservoir of smallpox remained, and it was in Asia.

In 1972 an extensive area still heavily endemic with smallpox stretched from Bangladesh through northern India and Nepal into Pakistan. Here case detection was inadequate and reporting systems were archaic; the importance of surveillance and containment was not appreciated, and when containment was attempted, it was usually done poorly. Support for the program by health authorities was lukewarm; so many efforts to control smallpox had failed over so many years that the disease was widely considered inevitable and its elimination impossible.

During the 1972–1973 smallpox season in India a WHO epidemiologist, tracing the source of infection of a case in the southern state of Andhra Pradesh, followed the trail into an adjacent state that was thought to be smallpox-free. There in one district he discovered a major epidemic. It had been known to district health workers but had been concealed. Rapid containment was crucial, but that required the prompt detection of all cases throughout a district of two million people. All available health personnel were mobilized for a house-to-house search,

which was two weeks in preparation and one week in execution. It revealed numerous previously undisclosed cases in addition to those recently discovered. Containment vaccination around each outbreak eliminated smallpox from the district within weeks. The experience underscored the danger of poor reporting, but it also showed what could be gained by a thorough search and demonstrated that vast numbers of health workers were deployed in India and could be mobilized quickly. Plans were made to undertake the same kind of search throughout India.

In October, 1973, the smallpox-eradication program in India conducted the first of a series of week-long searches that were scheduled once a month and involved more than 100,000 health workers. The results of the first search were ominous. The state of Uttar Pradesh, with a population of 90 million, had regularly been reporting from 100 to 300 cases of smallpox per week. The first one-week search in the state found more than 7,000 cases. And that was not all: a later assessment showed that only half of the villages officially reported as having been searched had actually been visited.

After that the techniques of case search were steadily improved. Between search weeks special surveillance teams asked questions at markets and in schools to uncover rumors of cases. A reward was offered to anyone who reported a case of smallpox and to the health worker receiving the report (see Figure 5.8). As the incidence of smallpox declined the amount of the reward was increased, always with extensive publicity. Containment measures were tightened. Special books were prepared in which every person in an infected village and for one mile around it was listed. Guards hired locally were stationed day and night at the homes of smallpox patients to keep the patient from leaving and to see to it that all visitors were vaccinated.

As case detection and notification improved, the number of reported cases climbed steeply. More than 218,000 cases were reported in India in 1974, the highest total recorded since 1958. Some newspapers called it a disaster, and more than one wrote an obituary of the global eradication program. Those involved in the program, however, felt that in the search tactic they had at last the key to smallpox eradication on the subcontinent.

In June, 1974, a new unit of measurement was adopted: the "infected village." A village (or a

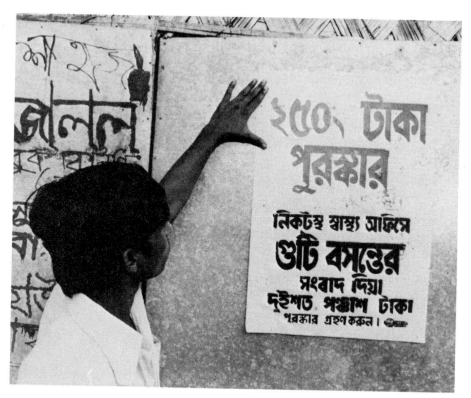

Figure 5.8 WALL POSTER IN BANGLADESH announcing a reward for reporting a smallpox case. The Bengali writing offers a "250-taka prize" (about $17) to anyone who reports a smallpox case to a health office. Reports and even rumors of cases were followed up by health workers.

ward in a city) was listed as infected if even one case was reported there; it remained on the list until six weeks after the onset of the last case and until an epidemiologist had certified (after a special search) that transmission had been stopped. The epidemic in India peaked in July, 1974, at which time there were more than 7,000 infected villages. The number fell steadily until in November it reached 350, but then the decline stopped. That caused concern because a new postmonsoon season with more rapid transmission of infection was beginning. Additional epidemiologists joined the fight, containment was made more rigid and in January the incidence of smallpox again began to decrease. May 24, 1975, saw the onset of the last known case of smallpox in India (see Figure 5.9).

Afghanistan had become smallpox-free in 1972, and Pakistan's last case was in October, 1974. Nepal, plagued by importations from India, recorded its last case in April, 1975. Bangladesh proved to be more difficult. There was great optimism late in 1974, when the number of infected villages in the country declined to only 91. Unfortunately nearly all the infected areas were in a region struck by famine after the most devastating floods in decades. Thousands of infected refugees began moving through Bangladesh, and in spite of heroic efforts it was impossible to stem the spread of disease. (In two days in one marketplace one beggar infected 52 people from 18 villages.) A further blow came in January of 1975, when slums in Dacca, the capital city, were bulldozed and about 500,000 people were displaced. Many of these people, some of them infected with smallpox, fanned out through the country, producing dozens of satellite outbreaks; the number of infected villages rose to a peak of 1,208 in late April. Then, under a presidential directive, a national emergency program was launched and the number of infected villages decreased sharply and steadily. On October 16, 1975,

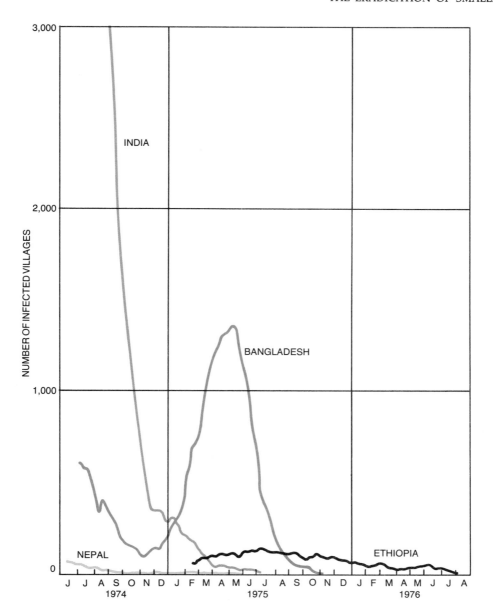

Figure 5.9 FINAL STAGES of eradication campaigns in the last four endemic countries were monitored by a weekly count of "infected villages," defined as those reporting a case within the past six weeks. The countdown was instituted in Ethiopia only early in 1975 and it was not until the summer of that year that it was considered to represent a reasonably complete national total.

the onset of the last case in Bangladesh was reported. The patient, three-year-old Rahima Banu, was the world's last known case of the severe form of smallpox (see Figure 5.4), variola major. After that 12,000 health workers supervised by nearly 100 epidemiologists repeatedly searched Bangladesh house by house. They found no cases, and it is unlikely that any more will be discovered, but surveillance will continue for two years.

There has been some concern that smallpox, after

having been declared eradicated, might emerge again from an unknown animal reservoir, from dormant virus in old scabs or from some other source. The most impressive evidence against the likelihood of such recurrence is the fact that for nine years no cases of smallpox have been discovered in the vast areas that have been smallpox-free, except for those imported from known endemic areas. Although 20 cases of an illness closely resembling smallpox have been detected in regions of Africa declared smallpox-free, in each such case "monkeypox" virus has been isolated, or identified by antibodies in victims' blood serum, as the causative factor. The reservoir of monkeypox is not known, but it is probably among rodents rather than monkeys. The disease is related to smallpox but is caused by a different virus, and its capacity for spreading from one human being to another appears to be almost nil.

What of the cost of the 10-year campaign? Approximately $83 million has been spent in international assistance for the smallpox-eradication program since 1967. The endemic countries themselves have spent roughly twice that amount, but few of them have spent much more than they were already spending on smallpox control. The total amount of money spent in international assistance is little more than half what was computed in 1968 to be the yearly expenditure for smallpox control in the U.S. alone; worldwide expenditures for smallpox vaccination and quarantine measures have been estimated as being in the range of from $1 billion to $2 billion a year. With the eradication of the disease smallpox vaccination will no longer be required, nor will international certificates of smallpox vaccination. Apart from the alleviation of human suffering, the savings have already repaid the small investment many times over.

The eradication of smallpox represents a major milestone in the history of medicine. It has demonstrated what can be achieved when governments throughout the world join an international organization in a common purpose. In perspective, however, the campaign must be seen as representing only a small first step toward achieving a tolerable level of public health throughout the world.

A logical next step would be to apply what has been learned in this campaign to immunization programs for controlling diphtheria, whooping cough, tetanus, measles, poliomyelitis and tuberculosis. Effective vaccines are available for all these diseases, but there has been little immunization outside the developed world. Now a number of the developing countries, given the confidence of achievement and recognizing how much can be accomplished with very little, have embarked on new immunization programs. With such campaigns one begins to see a perceptible—although far from adequate—shift from curative medicine for the rich to preventive medicine for all. Some of the difficulties of replicating the smallpox experience with other diseases are discussed in Chapter 6, "Obstacles to Developing Vaccines for the Third World."

POSTSCRIPT

The story of the eradication of smallpox is one of the most uplifting stories in human history. It illustrates what can be done when humanitarian instincts are allowed to flourish. Although this can truly be called "Jenner's legacy," it would not have happened as a result of standard medical practice. The eradication of smallpox required the tireless and devoted efforts of a vast army of public-health workers in numerous countries throughout the world. It is without question the towering achievement of the World Health Organization. The eradication of smallpox should silence those who are prone to criticize the United Nations.

Smallpox is a disease admirably suited for control by vaccination. By the middle of the 20th century, smallpox vaccination was completely routine in most of the developed countries of the world. Control of the disease in such countries by vaccination and quarantine had shown what could be done if sufficient will were exercised. In most Western countries, immigration authorities insisted that travelers show evidence of smallpox vaccination in order to be admitted to the country. Schoolchildren were routinely vaccinated, and the disease only arose if an isolated population, unvaccinated perhaps for religious reasons, became infected by introduction into such a population of an isolated infected individual. Such incidents were so rare as to be newsworthy.

In the underdeveloped parts of the world the situation was quite different. Smallpox was endemic and infected individuals might be found anywhere. Because the smallpox vaccine was so highly effective and so easily administered, an eradication campaign could be considered. All that would be necessary would be sufficient money for personnel, travel and supplies. Considering the amount of money spent by countries on military matters, the cost of the eradication program was quite modest. Through the combined contributions of the major world powers, the money was forthcoming and the campaign was a success.

The techniques used to contain and eradicate smallpox could, perhaps, be applied to other diseases, but with no other disease will success be so likely. The severity of smallpox, the effectiveness of the vaccine, its ease of administration and the characteristic symptoms that can be recognized even by someone without formal medical training make smallpox a unique case. For most diseases that are common in the Third World, we would probably be satisfied with a drastic reduction in incidence rather than complete eradication. The special problems of developing vaccination procedures for Third World countries are discussed in the next chapter.

Obstacles to Developing Vaccines for the Third World

Six vaccines are already in use there. Many others could be produced within 10 years. Yet those who have the know-how to make the needed vaccines have lacked incentives to apply it.

. . .

Anthony Robbins and Phyllis Freeman
November, 1988

Global immunization programs sponsored by the United Nations have made astonishing strides in the developing world during the past 25 years. Unfortunately this rapid forward movement is in danger of stalling. The loss of momentum would be tragic, given what has been achieved so far. The programs totally eradicated smallpox (see Chapter 5, "The Eradication of Smallpox") and have significantly reduced the annual death and disability caused by six major diseases: measles (which still kills two million children in the Third World every year), diphtheria, pertussis (whooping cough), tetanus, polio and tuberculosis. In 1974 an estimated 5 percent of the children in the developing world were being immunized against those six diseases; today, thanks to the World Health Organization's Expanded Program on Immunization (EPI), almost 50 percent of the children are completely immunized—that is, they receive all recommended doses of all six vaccines (see Figure 6.1). The EPI's aim is to reach every child by 1990.

Yet much remains to be done. In particular, new or improved vaccines are needed for the many other infectious diseases that cause unnecessary death and disability in the developing world, where four out of five children live. Children are the prime target of vaccination programs because they are the chief victims of infectious diseases. In Africa, Asia and Latin America acute respiratory infections (such as the pneumonias caused by *Streptococcus pneumoniae* and *Hemophilus influenzae* type b bacteria and by parainfluenza and respiratory syncytial viruses) and diarrheal diseases (such as infections caused by rotavirus and by *Shigella, Vibrio cholerae* and certain types of *Escherichia coli* bacteria) annually kill some eight million children under the age of five. These infections combine with other diseases, notably measles, malaria, tetanus, meningitis and typhoid fever, to kill an estimated 14 million children younger than five every year and to disable many millions more.

Strangely enough, it is not a lack of scientific know-how that is impeding the development of the needed vaccines. Many are already on the drawing

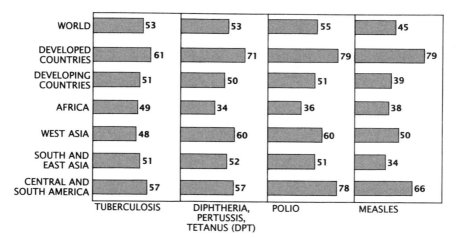

Figure 6.1 PERCENT OF INFANTS (up to a year old) in various parts of the world who in 1986 were receiving all prescribed doses of the EPI's vaccines against tuberculosis, diphtheria, pertussis (whooping cough), tetanus, polio and measles was estimated recently by UNICEF. The figure has been redrawn from one in UNICEF's *State of the World's Children 1988* and is based on data supplied by the WHO, UNICEF and the Population Division of the UN; it excludes China, where vaccination rates are generally higher than elsewhere in the developing world. In 1974 fewer than 5 percent of children were thought to be receiving all doses of all six vaccines. Today some 50 percent are completely immunized.

board in laboratories around the world. Indeed, in 1986 the Institute of Medicine of the U.S. National Academy of Sciences identified 19 priority infections for which, from a scientific standpoint, new or vastly improved vaccines could feasibly be produced by 1996 (see Figure 6.2).

Rather, the obstacles to the testing, mass production and distribution of the needed vaccines are economic and political. The UN is not equipped to produce the vaccines, and the handful of manufacturers—most of them in the developed world—that have the technological skill and production capacity needed for making human vaccines have little interest in that task.

During the past four years we have reviewed the vaccination needs of the Third World and have conferred with public health officials in many developing nations as well as with leaders of the EPI and most of the world's vaccine manufacturers. Our survey indicates that the current dilemma can be resolved. The solution requires, however, that the public and those involved in vaccine development and procurement gain a full understanding of why the EPI has been successful in the past, what the current challenges are and where there is room for cooperation between those who have and those who need.

Although finding a way to produce and deliver the vaccines required by the Third World will not be easy, it must be done. Vaccination programs are less expensive, easier to implement and sometimes more effective than other public health approaches now being pursued to varying degrees. For example, one could prevent many infectious diseases by controlling the factors that promote their spread, such as a high prevalence of disease-carrying insects (vectors), overcrowded living conditions and unsanitary sources of water for drinking and cooking. Yet vector-control programs, including those aimed at eliminating the mosquitoes that carry malaria, often are not completely successful. Moreover, many countries cannot yet afford the capital investment needed to improve housing, sanitation and drinking-water purity.

Relying on the delivery of effective treatments to the Third World is similarly problematic. Such drugs as antibiotics are highly effective against certain diseases or their secondary complications, for instance against shigellosis (which results in an estimated 650,000 deaths per year, primarily in children) and against the bacterial infections that often accompany infection by the respiratory syncytial virus. In addition oral rehydration therapy, which replaces the fluids and salts lost in diarrhea, is an

PATHOGEN	POTENTIAL EFFECTS	CASES PER YEAR (AND DEATHS)	INDUSTRIAL DEMAND
Dengue virus	Fever, shock, internal bleeding	35,000,000 (15,000*)	Small, (travelers to endemic areas)
Intestinal-toxin-producing *Escherichia coli* bacteria	Watery diarrhea, dehydration	630,000,000 (775,000*)	Small
Hemophilus influenzae type b bacterium	Meningitis, epiglottal swelling, pneumonia	800,000 (145,000*)	Great
Hepatitis A virus	Malaise, anorexia, vomiting, jaundice	5,000,000 (14,000)	Small
Hepatitis B virus	Same as hepatitis A; Chronic cirrhosis or cancer of liver	5,000,000 (822,000)	Moderate
Japanese encephalitis virus	Encephalitis, meningitis	42,000 (7,000*)	Small (travelers)
Mycobacterium leprae	Leprosy	1,000,000 (1,000)	None
Neisseria meningitidis bacterium	Meningitis	310,000 (35,000*)	Some (during epidemics)
Parainfluenza viruses	Bronchitis, pneumonia	75,000,000 (125,000*)	Great
Plasmodium protozoa	Malaria (with anemia, systemic inflammation)	150,000,000 (1,500,000*)	Moderate (travelers)
Rabies virus	Always-fatal meningitis and encephalitis	35,000 (35,000*)	Small
Respiratory syncytial virus	Repeated respiratory infections, pneumonia	65,000,000 (160,000*)	Great
Rotavirus	Diarrhea, dehydration	140,000,000 (873,000*)	Great
Salmonella typhi bacterium	Typhoid fever (with platelet and intestinal damage possible)	30,000,000 (581,000*)	Small (travelers)
Shigella bacteria	Diarrhea, dysentery, chronic infections	250,000,000 (654,000*)	None
Streptococcus Group A bacterium	Throat infection, then rheumatic fever, kidney disease	3,000,000 (52,000*)	Small
Streptococcus pneumoniae bacterium	Pneumonia, meningitis, serious inflammation of middle ear	100,000,000 (10,000,000*)	Small to moderate
Vibrio cholerae bacterium	Cholera (with diarrhea, dehydration)	7,000,000 (122,000*)	Small (travelers)
Yellow fever	Fever, jaundice, kidney damage, bleeding	85,000 (9,000*)	Small (travelers)

Figure 6.2 PATHOGENS identified by the Institute of Medicine of the U.S. National Academy of Sciences as ones for which vaccines could feasibly be developed and licensed by 1996. The number of cases and deaths due to each pathogen are estimated based on the institute's 1986 report, *New Vaccine Development, Establishing Priorities.* The asterisk indicates diseases for which children account for roughly half of the deaths or more. Virtually all deaths from dengue fever, parainfluenza, respiratory syncytial virus, rotavirus and pneumococcal meningitis occur in children. Two kinds of vaccines are already being made for hepatitis B.

inexpensive and easy way to counter many diarrheal diseases; it is necessary only to mix the contents of a prefilled packet with boiled water and feed the solution to the child.

Yet antibiotics and various other drugs are expensive, in part because many more doses are required than is the case with vaccines. Furthermore, the medical-care services that are necessary to identify sick children, make laboratory diagnoses and provide appropriate treatment have yet to be established in many developing nations. Also missing in many areas are massive public-education programs that could teach families to apply therapies that require little medical skill, such as oral rehydration therapy.

In the developed countries, infectious diseases for which effective vaccines have not been available have been controlled by improved public-health measures, such as water purification and sanitation. Yet, such public-health measures are often impossible in the Third World (see Figure 6.3).

The difficulty of implementing vector-control, sanitation, housing and treatment programs highlights another reason increasing the range of vaccines available to the Third World is an attractive approach to decreasing death and disability: an infrastructure—the EPI—is already being built for delivering vaccines to children. The infrastructure could readily be called on to deliver new vaccines for additional diseases. In the future the same infrastructure can also be extended to support other services that are important to child survival, such as family planning.

How has the EPI attained its impressive successes, and why can it not expand its vaccine arsenal by simply following the same strategy? To answer the first question, the EPI has been successful in part because, after some initial duplication of effort, the WHO has collaborated closely with the United Nations Children's Fund (UNICEF), which has a history of serving children in the developing world (see Figure 6.4). Together the organizations have helped the public-health authorities in the participating nations to set up systems for obtaining equipment,

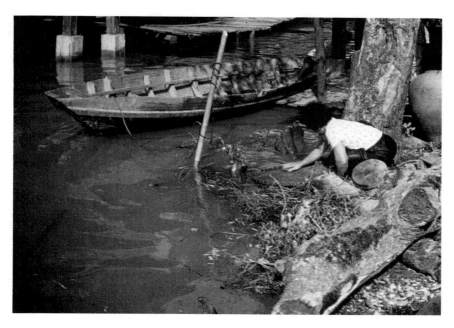

Figure 6.3 WATERWAY in East Pakistan has been identified as a source of cholera. Throughout the developing world, water taken for drinking or cooking from lakes, streams and rivers contaminated by body wastes facilitates the spread of cholera and such diseases as hepatitis, rotavirus, shigellosis and typhoid fever. Poor sanitation, over-crowding and an abundance of disease-carrying insects also promote disease. Programs to purify drinking-water supplies, improve sanitation and living conditions and eliminate vector populations can prevent much disease. For the short term, the expansion of immunization programs is the least expensive and easiest way to save lives.

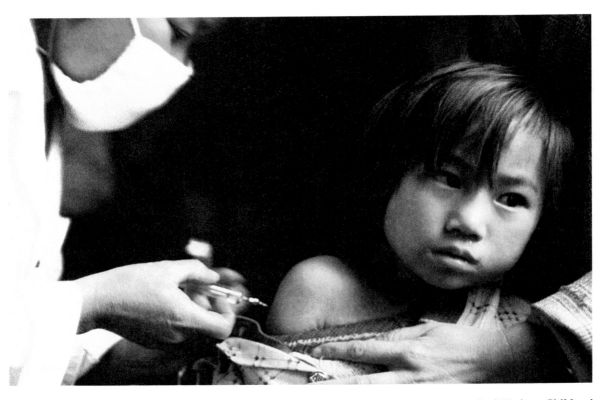

Figure 6.4 CHILD BEING IMMUNIZED in China is one of millions in the developing nations who have been protected against six dangerous infectious diseases as part of the United Nation's Expanded Program on Immunization (EPI). The participating agencies, including the World Health Organization and the United Nations Children's Fund (UNICEF), hope to also provide new or improved vaccines against many other pathogens that pose a major threat in the Third World.

training the personnel needed for vaccine delivery and ensuring that vaccines reach their destination in good order. These two UN agencies have been further supported since 1984 by the World Bank, the UN Development Program and the Rockefeller Foundation. In 1984 all five organizations formed the Task Force for Child Survival to bolster funding for and increase the stability of the EPI's global immunization activities.

The administrators of the EPI also found a way to obtain vaccines at unusually low prices: they chose vaccines that had been sold in the developed world for many years. The manufacturers had long since recouped their research and development costs, and so they could consider selling their products at close to the cost of production. We limit the use of the word research to the discovery of a candidate vaccine. Development is the costly and time-consum-

ing effort that includes producing small but high-quality batches of a candidate vaccine for testing, running clinical trials to demonstrate safety and effectiveness and to determine appropriate doses, meeting licensing requirements and generating the capacity to produce large, quality-controlled batches for mass distribution. It is at the development stage that many promising vaccines become stalled.

Having recouped its investment does not necessarily lead a company to sell its products at cost, but several corporations and public institutes have been willing to do so for any of a number of reasons. For some manufacturers, such as the government-owned National Institute of Public Health and Environmental Protection in the Netherlands, the reasons include a long-standing commitment to public health; those manufacturers do not expect to earn a profit from vaccines sold either domestically or abroad. Socialist nations that take part also commonly do so for humanitarian reasons and, as can be true for all participating manufacturers, to enhance their image in the developing world. For commercial firms, recognition and appreciation for their role in the EPI can facilitate other business activities, such as the sale of more profitable pharmaceuticals or the purchase of raw materials.

Many manufacturers also cooperate because they find the enterprise profitable. Selling large quantities of longstanding vaccines to the EPI can be remunerative even if the selling price is relatively low, because manufacturers who have the capacity to produce more vaccine than they sell at home or in other markets in the industrialized world realize economies of scale. These manufacturers can increase their production and do quality-control tests with existing personnel and equipment, thereby lowering the cost of each unit of vaccine produced. By selling vaccines to the EPI at close to cost, they recover a substantial fraction of their production costs and earn a greater profit on the higher-priced packages they sell in commercial markets.

Commercial wisdom holds that it is inefficient to produce a vaccine for a population base of fewer than 40 million. As a result certain manufacturers whose domestic markets are small, such as Smith Kline RIT of Belgium, have even been willing to expand their production capacity in order to win the EPI's business and so optimize production efficiency.

Although the EPI was able to capitalize on the varying motivations of many vaccine manufacturers to obtain low prices before 1983, in that year it managed to reduce its costs even more by initiating a bidding system. In particular, UNICEF, which buys most of the vaccines administered in Africa and some of those administered in Asia, and the Pan American Health Organization (PAHO), which buys vaccines for Latin America, solicit bids for the individual vaccines from several manufacturers and contract with the lowest qualified bidders. (The WHO itself now focuses more on science, administration and the training of personnel than on obtaining vaccines.)

Since the inception of the bidding program, all the interested manufacturers have been situated in Canada, Europe and Japan. The domestic market in the U.S. is so large that pharmaceutical firms here feel little need to compete elsewhere or to work with the EPI. They have also been discouraged from selling vaccines to the EPI at low cost because Congress has criticized them for not offering similarly low prices in their own backyard.

In 1988 the bidding system is enabling UNICEF and PAHO to buy vaccines at the extraordinarily low average price of five cents a dose, which translates into a cost of about 50 cents for the purchase of all doses of all six vaccines. The EPI spends more than 10 times as much per child on nonvaccine items: transportation, the personnel administering the vaccines and refrigeration equipment that protects the vaccine in a "cold chain."

The current procurement system, then, dealing as it does with long-used vaccines, emphasizes buying surplus goods. It takes advantage of all available incentives for makers to sell their products at, near or even below the marginal cost of production. The system continues to be highly successful and—once the delivery systems are fully in place —should enable the EPI to meet the goal of delivering the six current vaccines to all the children of the world. At that point the EPI will provide more than one billion doses per year.

The current program does face challenges. The EPI and the Task Force for Child Survival are concentrating on solving the problems of how to make inroads into areas where children are not yet receiving the six existing vaccines and how to ensure that vaccines continue to be delivered to each new generation of children after coverage is finally established worldwide. The EPI also constantly confronts the threat of rising prices. Moreover, existing vaccines have some shortcomings. For example, they lose potency when they are exposed to heat, which is a risk in developing countries, where refrigeration is often inadequate. The EPI badly needs vaccines that are heat-stable and ones that would increase the effectiveness and efficiency of the program in other ways, such as a measles vaccine that can be administered at or soon after birth to provide earlier protection.

The further problem of how to provide additional vaccines received little attention until recently, and yet it is crucial. Indeed, it is where creative thinking and new strategies are now needed the most. Not only would new vaccines save countless lives but also their availability would help to sustain the enthusiasm of political leaders in the developing nations for establishing the systems needed to meet the EPI's goals of providing every child with vaccines and maintaining high levels of coverage.

The UN has not totally ignored the problem of

new vaccines. The WHO does sponsor research into the creation and testing of new vaccines against infectious diseases in the developing world through five different programs based in Geneva. The programs influence vaccine research all through the world. Yet in 1987 the WHO's combined budget for vaccine research and development was only $10 million per year, much less than the $30 to $50 million the U.S. Institute of Medicine estimates is needed to develop a single vaccine.

The obstacles to the development and distribution of the needed vaccines are many, but among the most important is the fact that the decision to develop new vaccines is left almost entirely in the hands of a few institutes or commercial manufacturers in the developed world. The engineering knowledge and skills are concentrated in these few institutes and firms, several of which have already chosen not to participate in the EPI. Commercial manufacturers in particular cater to the needs of the prosperous, industrialized nations and find it necessary to recover development costs before considering selling their products at close to the cost of production.

For instance, vaccine producers in the U.S., Canada, Western Europe and Japan are focusing a great deal of attention on improving the diphtheria-pertussis-tetanus (DPT) vaccine's pertussis component, which in rare instances causes seizures or brain damage. A new vaccine is certain to be expensive — from 10 to 100 times the current price to the EPI. The extra expense, if the EPI could afford it, would not increase the vaccine's efficacy, reach new populations or offer protection against new diseases.

In spite of this bleak picture, the old strategy of waiting for research and development costs to be recovered and then buying in bulk at a steep discount may still work for those vaccines that have a large market in the developed world or that have some market for travelers. There may be a long wait, however. When new vaccines come on the market, they tend to be expensive, not only because of the need to recoup standard development costs but also because new — and hence costly — technologies have often been employed to produce them. The new technologies are not always crucial. Many times they are chosen in preference to an older technology because they may result in a vaccine that has somewhat fewer side effects or is slightly more effective, but they often do so at the public health cost of making the product inaccessible to the Third World.

One product that is already on the market is a vaccine against hepatitis B. In fact, there are two types of hepatitis B vaccines: both consist of antigens (fragments of an organism that elicit the production of protective antibodies) from the virus, but one type is produced by genetic engineering and the other is made with an older technology that relies on isolating antigens from the blood plasma of infected individuals. The price of one such plasma-based vaccine, made in Korea with a technique developed in New York, is now about $1. This is still eight times costlier than the most expensive vaccine (measles) now bought by the EPI, but if the vaccine meets the WHO's standards of safety and efficacy, it may be adopted by the EPI as it waits for the prices of the potentially superior genetically engineered vaccines to drop significantly. The first of the genetically engineered vaccines to be licensed in the U.S. costs as much as $130 for a three-dose series.

Vaccines for AIDS and rotavirus, which are under intensive study because the diseases affect many people in the industrialized nations, may also become available in the future and affordable sometime later. A malaria vaccine too seems possible, since the demand from travelers living in industrial countries may well combine with the very large population exposed in the Third World to encourage commercial development. Other vaccines that may meet the needs of a smaller subset of travelers (those against dengue virus and hepatitis A infections, for instance) are less likely to be produced or, if they are produced, to be affordable to the Third World.

The waiting strategy will certainly not make available vaccines that have no market in the industrial world. As things stand now, several important vaccines that are scientifically feasible, according to the Institute of Medicine, are likely to be neglected by commercial firms for lack of a market in the industrialized nations. Such vaccines include ones against shigellosis, leprosy and infections caused by *Streptococcus pneumoniae* (in infants) and enterotoxigenic *E. coli* (*E. coli* that produce intestinal toxins). The same may be true for improved versions of the vaccines for measles, polio, cholera, typhoid, Japanese encephalitis and yellow fever.

Thus market forces militate against the production of critically needed vaccines for the Third World, and even the vaccines that have a chance of being produced are for the most part unlikely to be affordable any time soon, if ever. In some cases the EPI may have to consider buying potentially inferior products (such as the plasma-based vaccine for hepatitis B instead of a genetically engineered one) because they are the least costly. Even that option is not always open: manufacturers who have employed relatively low-cost technologies to make vaccines may remove their less expensive products from the market when they introduce versions made with a more advanced technology.

The situation is discouraging but not beyond redemption. Indeed, at least four approaches are worth considering. In one approach, which essentially accepts the status quo, the UN would raise the money to buy vaccines at close to their market price (in other words, a price that includes development costs and profits) in the hope that the promise of a new, lucrative market would encourage the industry to make the needed investment in development. For this approach to be successful the EPI would have to predict the number of doses it would buy, something that could probably be done. On the negative side, UNICEF and PAHO would have to commit themselves to buying given quantities at top dollar for a long time—a commitment they probably could not make.

A second option is for the UN to create a public institute to develop and manufacture its own vaccines, bypassing commercial makers. If the institute were equipped with advanced technology and staffed by the finest epidemiologists, molecular biologists, fermentation engineers and other professionals from around the world, it might well produce rapid results.

Such an institute could pursue new technologies that are particularly appropriate to Third World public-health needs without having to earn rapid profits. For example, workers might be able to insert genes for antigens from different bacteria and viruses into a single carrier organism—such as the vaccinia virus that once constituted the smallpox vaccine or the bacillus Calmette-Guérin (BCG), which is used as the vaccine against tuberculosis—to produce a single vaccine capable of eliciting immunity to a wide range of infections. The institute staff might also be able to advance the development of stable cocktails, or mixtures, of antigens that would immunize against several diseases at the same time, thereby improving the ability of the developing countries to provide complete coverage for their children.

As the UN's health programs expand, the possibility that the organization could operate such an institute increases, but the disadvantages of the solution are as tangible as its appeal. The creation of such a center would be both costly and time-consuming, and the politics of international cooperation are brutal. The difficulty the UN Industrial Development Organization (UNIDO) has had in establishing two new biotechnology centers is instructive. In the first five years not a single product has been put forward. Success in vaccine development and production is too critical to the health of the world to rely at the start on an international center alone.

A third alternative is to establish development and production units in countries or regions of the Third World with large populations. Such units would be dedicated to creating, developing and producing vaccines against the diseases that are most prevalent or destructive in the region. The concept is likely to appeal to the participating nations of the EPI, which are eager to develop new technologies. Funding for the transfer of technology is also a traditional development activity and might attract money that would otherwise not be available for vaccination programs.

A major roadblock to this alternative is the fact that the World Bank and other agencies that might provide loans to establish such units are increasingly concerned with meeting banker's standards (seeing a good return on an investment) when they finance new industrial enterprises. The development and production of vaccines to meet the health needs of the Third World is unlikely to turn a profit.

Even if financing can be obtained, the full benefits of this approach will take years to realize. It will take time for any institute to produce a product, time for the institute to address the range of needs in its region and more time still until a network of such institutes can meet all the vaccination needs of every region in the developing world.

The idea is nonetheless worth trying as a long-term strategy, and actually it is being pursued on a small scale by PAHO and the Rockefeller Foundation. Convinced that the aim of investment in regional vaccine production should be advances in public health and science rather than financial gain, PAHO and the Rockefeller Foundation are exploring the creation of one or more centers for developing and producing vaccines in Latin America. If the centers are successful in demonstrating that otherwise competitive nations can cooperate to solve a regional health problem, international-aid organizations may decide to help establish similar centers in Africa and Asia.

There is a fourth approach, which seems to us to be a rapid and short-term strategy for obtaining tangible results before the end of this century. As in the first alternative, the UN would raise money to pay manufacturers, but the funds would be earmarked specifically for the development of particular vaccines deemed important for large parts of the Third World. For many of the same reasons that now lead manufacturers to take part in the EPI, the institutes and companies that develop the products would then sell them to the EPI at or near the cost of production (with no development costs added on). The advantage of this approach over the first one is that a finite amount of money would have to be raised for each vaccine, and the EPI would receive a long-term commitment for a supply of vaccine at a low price.

Raising money for vaccine development is not out of the question. There are already mechanisms in place to fund vaccine research; for instance, the World Bank and the UN Development Program support such research. Those mechanisms would simply have to be extended or copied to support a program of vaccine development.

On the other hand, the UN and other agencies that run international-aid programs would have to make the difficult decision to spend money outside the Third World—in industrial nations, where most manufacturers with good track records in translating laboratory discoveries into full-scale production capacity are currently situated. This would be a necessary concession now, to ensure speedy, consistent and high-quality vaccine manufacture. With time, however, it should be possible to transfer much of the resulting technology to the developing nations so that they can build on any technology they have already acquired and make their own vaccines.

There are signs that the fourth approach may actually be tested soon. Key public and private manufacturers around the world have expressed some willingness to undertake the development and production of EPI vaccines on a contractual basis and then to sell the products at close to cost (although several manufacturers still express concern about whether the volume of purchases would be adequate). For some companies such an arrangement would be an attractive way to explore advanced technologies and have the needed tools subsidized.

There has also been some discussion at the UN of creating a revolving fund through which the development arm of the UN and other aid programs would pay the initial development costs. Under this plan UNICEF and PAHO would pay only the cost of production for the resulting vaccines and a small surcharge that would serve to replenish the fund so that more development could be pursued.

Actually any of the four approaches, or some combination of them, could succeed. The task now is to mobilize international agencies to confront directly and soon the lack of new vaccines, and to convince those who have the needed scientific knowledge and technical skill to apply such assets on behalf of all children—both in the developing nations and in the industrialized ones.

POSTSCRIPT

The countries of the world are often divided into three categories, those under U.S. influence, those under Soviet influence, and those called Third World countries that are unallied with either the U.S. or the Soviet. However, for public-health purposes it is more accurate to recognize only two groups of countries, developed and developing. Among developed countries we would include the U.S., most of the countries of Europe (including the U.S.S.R.) Japan, Australia, New Zealand and Israel. Developing countries would include most of the countries of Africa, Central America, South America and Asia. There is a sharp contrast in the degree of importance of infectious diseases as causes of death in developing versus developed countries. In developing regions of the world, infectious diseases account for between 30 and 50 percent of deaths, whereas infectious diseases account for less than 10 percent of deaths in developed countries. Diseases that were leading causes of death in the U.S. and Western Europe nearly a century ago, such as tuberculosis and gastroenteritis, are still leading causes of death in developing countries. Furthermore, the majority of deaths due to infectious disease in developing countries occur among infants and children. While in developed countries most deaths occur in individuals 65 years or older, in developing countries almost half of the deaths occur in youths under 14 years of age. Since the youth of a country is its future, this disparity in age at death is especially tragic. The economic cost of infectious disease to a developing country is vast. A small investment in control of infectious disease should result in a large economic return for society.

Although the health status of people in developing countries is due in part to general nutrient deficiencies that make individuals more susceptible to infection, it is also due to the lower levels of public-health protection, which make infection more likely in the first place. However, many developing countries are unable to expand food production and it is very expensive to institute public-health measures. Treatment of infections with antibiotics and other antimicrobial agents is also prohibitively expensive. Here is where vaccines can make their largest contribution. It is much cheaper to vaccinate than to treat; prevention is almost always cheaper than re.

But there are two major problems with introducing ccines into the Third World. The first is cost. Vacnes that are made by pharmaceutical companies in veloped countries are expensive because they rect the high research costs involved in their development. The second problem is availability. Many nfectious diseases rampant in the Third World are rare or absent in the developed countries, so that pharmaceutical companies have no economic motivation to carry out the necessary research. The authors of this chapter offer some hope that both these problems can be overcome. However, despite the difficulties, vaccines are being applied worldwide for six major diseases: measles, diphtheria, pertussis, tetanus, polio and tuberculosis.

The efforts to develop vaccines for the Third World emphasize again the crucial importance of the World Health Organization. Chapter 5, "The Eradication of Smallpox," discusses the central role of the WHO in that campaign. For other infectious diseases, the Expanded Program on Immunization of the WHO is playing the major role. It is indeed heartening that almost 50 percent of children in the developing countries are completely immunized against the six major diseases mentioned above. With continued effort, every child in the world should be reached in a few years.

Synthetic Vaccines

A short chain of amino acids assembled in the laboratory to mimic a site on the surface of a viral protein can give rise to antibodies of predetermined specificity that confer immunity against the virus.

. . .

Richard A. Lerner
February, 1983

Vaccination is one of man's most significant inventions (see Chapters 4, 5 and 6). It has eliminated smallpox and brought such diseases as diphtheria, poliomyelitis and measles under control. Yet the procedure remains imperfect: the safety of a vaccine cannot be absolutely ensured. Immunization against viral infection is achieved by injecting a virus that elicits antibodies capable of neutralizing the agent of a disease; the injected virus is not itself likely to cause infection because it has been either attenuated or killed. An attenuated virus is one whose virulence in human beings has been reduced by mutation in the course of passage through some different animal host, so that the virus becomes adapted to survival in that animal rather than in human beings. (The cowpox virus, which confers immunity to smallpox, is in effect a naturally attenuated virus.) An attenuated virus is, however, a living organism and therefore a changeable one. It can mutate further, possibly increasing in virulence. Even in the absence of mutation it may possibly have some unknown long-term effect comparable to those of slow-acting "latent" viruses. These possibilities are eliminated if the virus is killed and thereby inactivated, but there have been instances where an incompletely inactivated virus has caused disease.

Other problems are common to both attenuated-virus and killed-virus vaccines. Any facility where viruses are grown to make a vaccine is a reservoir from which an agent of disease can accidentally be disseminated. Moreover, because viruses replicate only in a living system, they are commonly grown in cultured cells or fertilized eggs or are isolated from the blood of infected animals (from infected human beings in the case of the virus causing hepatitis B); the cultured cells, eggs or blood may contain undetected substances, notably other viruses, that can contaminate the vaccine. Some vaccines, even some killed-virus ones, must be kept under refrigeration from the time they are prepared until they are inoculated, and maintaining a dependable "cold chain" can be a formidable problem in underdeveloped parts of the world.

For all these reasons there has been increasing interest in the preparation of synthetic vaccines, which is to say vaccines containing not intact viruses but merely peptides (short protein chains) that have been constructed in the laboratory to mimic a very small region of the virus's outer coat and that can nonetheless give rise to antibodies capable of neutralizing the virus. Experimental vaccines of this kind have now been developed in a number of laboratories. In the process much has been learned about the immunological structure of proteins; indeed, the ability to synthesize peptides that elicit antibodies of precise and predetermined specificity may give molecular biologists a battery of tools whose significance may rival the clinical significance of synthetic vaccines.

B efore reporting on experiments and results and on what we have learned about protein structure I should describe the immune system's mode of defense against viral infection. A virus is a small package of genetic information (DNA or RNA) enclosed in a capsid consisting of many copies of a protein or of several different proteins; the capsid may in turn be enveloped in a membrane studded with proteins. Infection begins when a specific site on the surface of the virus binds to a specific receptor on the surface of the cell. The virus penetrates the cell membrane and appropriates the cell's biosynthetic machinery to make many copies of itself, which burst out of the cell and go on to infect more cells (see Figure 7.1a). The infective process may be blocked by the immune system if the host has previously been exposed to the same virus or has been immunized against it with a vaccine. In either case certain of the immune-system cells called lymphocytes will have been primed to recognize the virus. When receptors on one of these lymphocytes encounter the virus, an immune response is triggered, one result of which is the proliferation of plasma cells that secrete antibodies against sites on the surface of the virus. The antibodies bind to those sites, coat the surface of the virus and block its attachment to receptors on cells. The virus is neutralized. (see Figure 7.1b).

The site that is recognized by a specific lymphocyte and to which the antigen-binding site of a specific antibody subsequently binds is called an antigenic determinant. It is usually a limited patch of a viral surface protein. That being the case, might it not be possible to elicit antibodies capable of neutralizing a virus by injecting as a vaccine peptides that constitute antigenic determinants (see Figure 7.1c)? The notion that a small part of an infectious agent might serve as a vaccine goes back more than 45 years, to studies done by Walther F. Goebel of the Rockefeller Institute for Medical Research. He showed that immunizing mice with a sugar chain

from the surface of the bacterium that causes pneumonia would protect the mice from subsequent infection. The feasibility of making immunogenic peptides to order was greatly increased in the 1960's when R. B. Merrifield of Rockefeller University developed a method for automatically linking amino acids, the subunits of proteins, to make a peptide.

It is not always easy to determine the amino acid sequence of a particular peptide in a large protein molecule, but a way around that difficulty was found. The amino acid sequence of a protein is specified by the sequence of the subunits called nucleotides in the nucleic acid (DNA or RNA) encoding the protein. One of the major accomplishments of biotechnology was the development of new techniques for determining the nucleotide sequence of DNA. Now it became possible to very rapidly determine the complete sequence of the DNA of a virus (or of a DNA copy of a viral RNA). Then, as shown in Figure 7.2, one could identify a nucleic acid sequence likely to encode a surface protein and translate that region according to the genetic code to derive the amino acid sequence of the protein. Then, exploiting Merrifield's procedure, one could synthesize short peptides in various regions of the protein, inject them into laboratory animals and see if they would give rise to antibodies that bind to the natural protein and perhaps neutralize the virus.

Before one could begin rationally designing vaccines, however, some difficult questions had to be answered having to do with the nature of an antigenic determinant and whether or not a short synthetic peptide could be expected to mimic one. Antibodies bind to protein sites by reason of shape and electric charge. The backbone of a protein is a chain of carbon and nitrogen atoms bristling with projections: the side chains of successive amino acids, each of which has a characteristic shape and array of charges. The sequence of the amino acids (which constitutes the primary structure of the protein) and their consequent short-range interactions determine how the chain twists locally into what is called the secondary structure: perhaps a helix or a sharp turn. Interactions among secondary structures in turn determine how the chain folds back on itself to form the complex tertiary structure characteristic of proteins.

It follows that there can be two kinds of antigenic determinant (see Figure 7.3). If the antigen-binding site of an antibody molecule recognizes and binds to an array of contiguous amino acid side chains, one

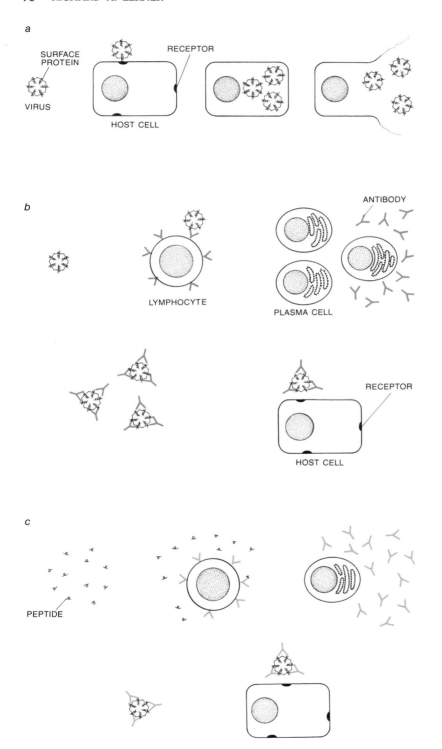

a

SURFACE PROTEIN

VIRUS

RECEPTOR

HOST CELL

b

ANTIBODY

LYMPHOCYTE

PLASMA CELL

RECEPTOR

HOST CELL

c

PEPTIDE

Figure 7.1 A VIRUS INFECTS A CELL (*a*) by attaching itself to a receptor on the cell, entering the cell and taking over the cell's machinery to make many copies of itself, which burst the cell. An attenuated or killed virus can be injected as a vaccine (*b*). When such a virus encounters a receptor on a lymphocyte that is genetically programmed to recognize and make antibody against a surface protein of the virus, the lymphocyte is stimulated to form a clone of antibody-secreting plasma cells. In any subsequent exposure to the virus the antibodies bind to the protein and neutralize the virus by blocking its attachment to host cells. A synthetic peptide mimicking part of the surface protein can serve as a vaccine (*c*). It too elicits antibodies able to bind to the surface protein and neutralize the virus.

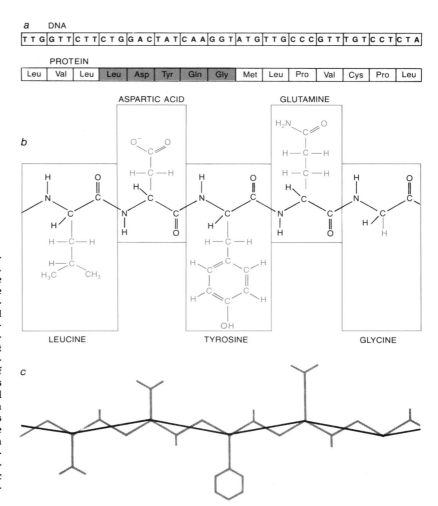

a DNA

| T T G | G T T | C T T | C T G | G A C | T A T | C A A | G G T | A T G | T T G | C C C | G T T | T G T | C C T | C T A |

PROTEIN

| Leu | Val | Leu | Leu | Asp | Tyr | Gln | Gly | Met | Leu | Pro | Val | Cys | Pro | Leu |

ASPARTIC ACID

GLUTAMINE

b

LEUCINE

TYROSINE

GLYCINE

c

Figure 7.2 NUCLEOTIDE SE-UENCE of a stretch of viral DNA encodes the amino acid sequence of a viral protein (*a*). Once the DNA sequence is known, investigators can predict the amino acid sequence and pick out for synthesis those peptides, or short segments of the protein chain, that seem likely to give rise to antibodies. The chemical structure of part of the peptide shown in *a* is diagrammed (*b*). Each amino acid is characterized by a side chain (*color*) that projects from what is called the alpha carbon. In the computer displays of proteins in this chapter either the alpha-carbon backbone is shown (*c*) in simplified form (*black*) or in atomic detail with hydrogen atoms excluded (*gray*).

speaks of a continuous antigenic determinant. A discontinuous determinant, on the other hand, is one made up of groups of amino acids that are separated from one another along the chain but are brought into proximity by tertiary folding.

For many years, a considerable body of immunological doctrine suggested that synthesized peptides were not likely to mimic the natural antigenic determinants of intact viral proteins. In the first place it appears that the immune response to a viral protein in the course of a natural infection is directed to a small number of antigenic determinants confined to a few parts of the protein molecule; specifically, there is evidence that a protein's immunogenicity

(its ability to elicit antibodies) is accounted for by only one site for every 50 amino acids. Moreover, most of these relatively few antigenic determinants seem to be discontinuous ones. To make a peptide simulating such a determinant one would have to make a long stretch of the protein; such a synthesis is technically feasible but inefficient. If a long peptide were synthesized, it seemed unlikely to fold itself into the correct tertiary structure in the absence of the rest of the molecule. Indeed, it was thought the individual side chains in a short peptide would not spontaneously orient themselves to mimic even the simpler secondary structure of a continuous determinant.

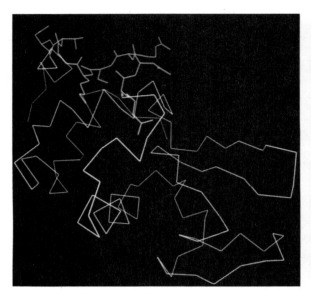 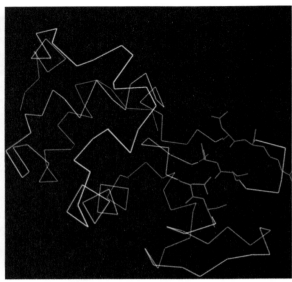

Figure 7.3 ANTIGENIC DETERMINANTS are sites on a protein that are recognized by antibodies and to which the antibodies bind. The two kinds of determinants are illustrated by these computer displays in which part of the main chain of the enzyme lysozyme, a typical antigen, is shown in yellow, with antigenic determinants (side chains included) picked out in orange. A continuous determinant *(left)* is one formed by an array of contiguous amino acids along one segment of the chain. A discontinuous determinant *(right)* is one composed of several segments that are separated from one another along the chain but are brought together to form a single site by the tertiary folding of the protein.

To challenge these rather pessimistic assumptions my colleagues and I at the Research Institute of Scripps Clinic decided to synthesize in short segments almost the entire length of a viral protein and see whether antibodies to many of the peptides might not react with the entire protein. The molecule we chose was the hemagglutinin of one strain of the influenza virus. The structure of the influenza hemagglutinin is shown in Figure 7.4. It is a glycoprotein (a protein with sugar chains attached) that forms spikes radiating from the spherical envelope of the virus. The hemagglutinin spikes have important functions. They mediate the binding of the virus to a host cell. As their name indicates, they cause red blood cells to clump together. And they are primarily responsible for eliciting antibodies that neutralize the virus.

Two factors made the influenza hemagglutinin an attractive choice for our studies. Walter Fiers of the State University of Ghent in Belgium and his colleagues had determined the nucleotide sequence of the gene encoding the protein, and from it they had predicted the amino acid sequence. Ian A. Wilson and Don C. Wiley of Harvard University and John J. Skehel of the National Institute for Medical Research in London had determined the structure of the protein by X-ray crystallography, so that we would be able to relate each peptide we synthesized to a particular region of the secondary and tertiary structure. A molecule of the hemagglutinin is composed of two protein chains designated HA1 and HA2; each spike is a trimer consisting of three such molecules. HA1 seems to be the primary target of the immune system, and so we turned first to that chain.

We synthesized 20 peptides accounting for some 75 percent of the length of the chain and sampling a wide variety of secondary and tertiary structures. (The procedure used to determine the antigenicity of the peptides is shown in Figure 7.5.) We injected each of the peptides, bound to a large carrier protein, into rabbits and tested serum from each rabbit (by what is called an enzyme-linked immunosorbent assay) for the presence of antibodies that would bind to the injected peptide, to the hemagglutinin molecule and to the intact virus. All 20 of

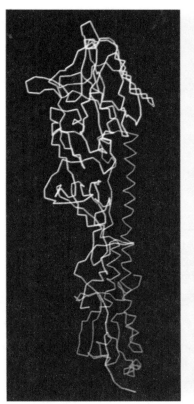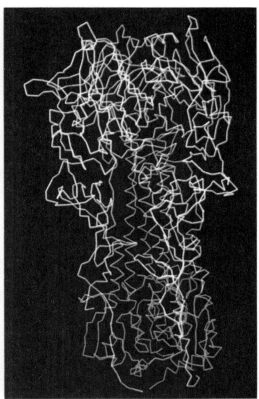

Figure 7.4 HEMAGGLUTININ MOLECULE of the influenza virus is made up of two protein chains, *HA*1 (*purple*) and *HA*2 (*orange*). The three-dimensional structure of the molecule (*left*) is based on X-ray crystallographic data supplied by Ian A. Wilson and Don C. Wiley of Harvard University and John J. Skehel of the National Institute for Medical Research in London; only the backbone is displayed. Three *HA*1 chains and three *HA*2 chains are associated in the hemagglutinin trimer (*right*). Trimers form spikes on the spherical envelope of the virus particle.

the peptides gave rise to antibodies against themselves; 15 of the antipeptide antibodies reacted with the protein molecule and 17 of them bound to the influenza virus. In other words, a peptide from almost any region of a viral protein can elicit an antibody that will recognize the entire protein, either in purified form or on the surface of the virus; the natural immunogenicity of a protein (the only kind that has been much studied up to now) is less than the potential immunogenicity of its parts. The only requirement seems to be that the synthesized peptide be on the surface of the folded protein, where the antibody can get at it.

There are a number of ways to estimate whether a given peptide is on the surface of a protein — or, to put it more exactly, whether a peptide (or part of it) is accessible to antibody molecules in solution in an animal's blood. One of the most precise ways is to program a computer to make a graphic display of the solvent-accessible regions (see Figure 7.6). First the peptide under study is displayed, complete with its branching side chains, in the conformation it assumes on the intact protein molecule. Then the computer rolls a sphere representing a water molecule around the peptide. The sphere penetrates where it can, given the van der Waals radius (loosely, the zone of influence in terms of electric charge) of the water molecule and of the atoms of the side chains. The sphere leaves a dot at each point of contact with the peptide, thus in effect drawing a map of the solvent-accessible regions of the peptide.

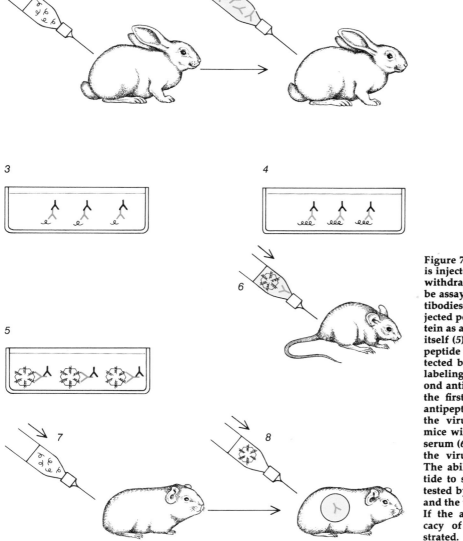

Figure 7.5 SYNTHETIC PEPTIDE is injected into a rabbit (*1*). Serum withdrawn from the rabbit (*2*) can be assayed for the presence of antibodies able to bind to the injected peptide (*3*), to the viral protein as a whole (*4*) and to the virus itself (*5*). The binding of the antipeptide antibody (*color*) is detected by noting the activity of a labeling enzyme coupled to a second antibody (*black*) that binds to the first one. The ability of the antipeptide antibody to neutralize the virus is tested by injecting mice with the virus and the antiserum (*6*); if the mouse stays well, the virus has been neutralized. The ability of the synthetic peptide to serve as a vaccine can be tested by injecting the peptide (*7*) and the virus (*8*) into a guinea pig. If the animal survives, the efficacy of the vaccine is demonstrated.

The scheme I have described is effective, but it does require that the structure of a virus and its proteins be known in atomic detail, and such data are not available for many viruses. Fortunately there is a way to predict which parts of a protein are likely to be on the surface if one knows only the amino acid sequence. The 20 amino acids can be characterized for the most part as being either hydrophilic (water-attracting) or hydrophobic (water-repelling). The hydrophobic amino acids are most often buried in the core of the folded protein, whereas the hydrophilic ones are usually on the outside of the molecule (see Figure 7.7). The four most hydrophilic amino acids are lysine, arginine, aspartic acid and glutamic acid. One simply assumes the regions of a protein that are relatively rich in these amino acids are likely to be exposed to an aqueous environment and therefore are on the surface.

Our results with the influenza virus suggested, as I pointed out above, that just about any surface peptide should give rise to antibodies able to react with the entire protein. How is it that a lone peptide can be depended on to assume a conformation similar to its conformation when it is folded into the complete protein molecule? It may be the very lack of constraints on shape that gives rise to the correct shape. An injected small peptide, in solution in an animal's bloodstream, keeps twisting and bending. As it changes shape it presumably continues to encounter lymphocytes, and hence to trigger the secretion of antibodies against each shape in turn. One of those shapes, it now seems clear, is likely to coincide closely with the conformation the peptide adopts as part of a large protein. (It is interesting to note that in many cases small peptides are more effective in eliciting antibodies against a viral protein than the purified protein is. Perhaps the isolated protein locks itself into a folded configuration that is different from the shape it assumes when it is arrayed with many copies of itself on a virus.)

If virtually any surface region of a viral protein can elicit antibodies against that protein, the way is open for designing a vaccine rationally instead of injecting whole virus particles and in effect taking whatever the immune system offers. That is being done in a number of laboratories. The first vaccine we developed was against the virus of foot-and-mouth disease, a historic plague of animals (cattle in particular) that is still a serious problem on every continent except Australia and North America. Some three billion doses of killed-virus vaccine are administered annually in an effort to control it. The virus shell is composed of 240 protein molecules, 60 copies each of the four viral proteins VP1, VP2, VP3 and VP4. There have been attempts to make a vaccine based on VP1, which is thought to be the major natural target of neutralizing antibody, but the entire protein has proved to be not very immunogenic. In collaboration with Fred Brown and David J. Rowlands of the Animal Virus Research Institute in England, we undertook to synthesize a more immunogenic subregion of the protein.

The sequence of VP1's 213 amino acids had already been determined from the nucleotide sequence. The structure of the protein is not yet known in atomic detail. Analysis of the amino acid sequence, however, was enough to draw our attention to the region between amino acids 141 and 160. The region is fairly rich in the hydrophilic side chains of arginine, lysine and aspartic acid, suggesting it might be on the surface. The amino acid proline is often found where a protein makes a sharp bend (which may make for immunological specificity), and the region has two prolines.

Most important, it was known that in this region the amino acid sequence undergoes considerable variation from strain to strain. A virus needs to evade a host's immune-system defenses long enough to invade host cells and produce progeny. It does so by continually changing the antigenic determinants on its outer shell or envelope, with the result that antibodies formed earlier against a parental strain will not bind to the altered virus and neutralize it. In less teleological terms, what happens is that natural selection encourages the survival of a strain in which spontaneous mutation has brought about an immunologically significant variation. A region subject to such mutation is likely to be one that ordinarily elicits antibodies, and so a peptide from that region is a good candidate for a synthetic vaccine.

We synthesized a number of peptides from the VP1 of the foot-and-mouth virus, including the peptide spanning positions 141 to 160, coupled each one to a carrier molecule and injected it into rabbits. After determining that the peptides elicited antibodies against themselves, we did a bioassay to test their ability to neutralize the virus. When the rabbit antiserum to peptide 141–160 was injected into mice along with the virus, it effectively neutralized the virus; the mice were given what is called passive immunity by the injected antipeptide antibody. There are three major strains of the foot-and-mouth virus; we had worked with type O. When we tested the same antibody's effect on the other two strains, the neutralization was much weaker, supporting the impression that changes in this particular region of VP1 allow the virus to elude antibodies made against a different strain.

The real test of any vaccine is its ability to confer not only passive immunity but also active immu-

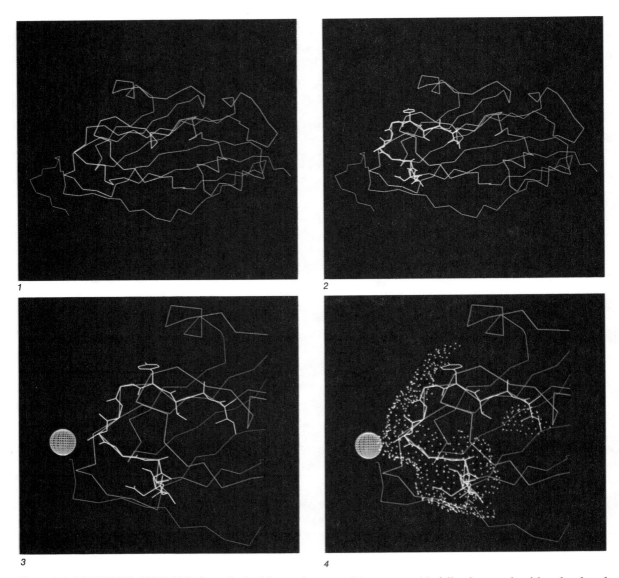

Figure 7.6 COMPUTER DISPLAYS show the backbone of the surface domain of the protein on the outer shell of the virus (1) based on coordinates determined by Stephen C. Harrison and colleagues. A single peptide of the protein is picked out in yellow, with the side chains of its component amino acids indicated in atomic detail (2). A sphere representing a water molecule is displayed (3), and the sphere is rolled around the peptide to generate a map of the surface accessible to water (4), following an algorithm developed by Michael L. Connolly. A similar dot surface map is generated to show what parts of the peptide are still accessible to water when three copies of the protein are associated in an array on the surface of the virus (5) and when four such arrays (out of 60) are in position on the outer surface of the virus (6).

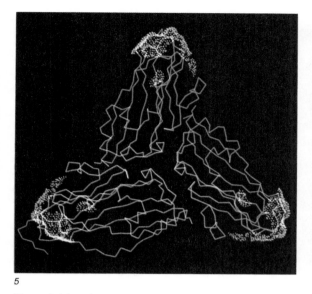

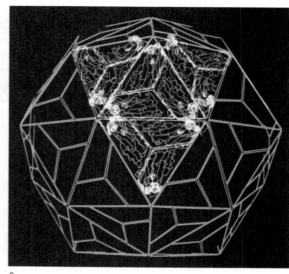

5

6

Figure 7.6 (continued).

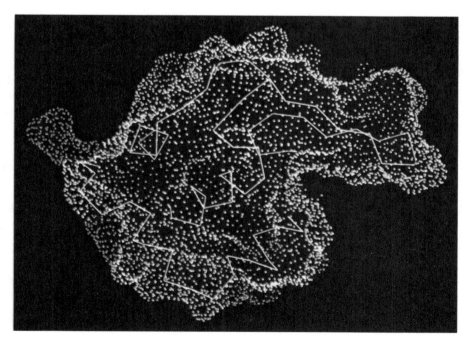

Figure 7.7 SOLVENT-ACCESSIBLE SURFACE of the lysozyme molecule is mapped by the method demonstrated in Figure 7.6, but with the dots color-coded according to the amino acid responsible for each part of the surface: orange for the basic amino acids lysine and arginine, green for the acidic ones aspartic acid and glutamic acid and blue for all others. The basic and acidic amino acids are the most hydrophilic (water-attracting) ones. As the display demonstrates, they tend to be exposed on the surface. If a protein's structure is not known in detail, one can simply assume peptides rich in hydrophilic amino acids will be immunogenic.

nity, that is, to cause the immune system to synthesize its own antibodies for protection against a future attack. We immunized guinea pigs with one shot (200 micrograms) of the synthetic-peptide vaccine and after 35 days administered a powerful dose of the virus: 10,000 times the dose normally required to infect half of a group of animals. None of the immunized animals came down with the disease, whereas all the unimmunized control animals did. A similar active-immunity test in cattle is now under way in England. Already we have found that cattle immunized with the peptide secrete antibody at a concentration that should protect them from a virus challenge.

A practical vaccine will, of course, have to protect against all three strains of the virus. We have synthesized peptides from the same region (141 to 160) of the VP1 of type-A and type-C viruses, which have slightly different amino acid sequences. So far antibodies to these peptides have been bioassayed in mice, and they do neutralize viruses of type A and type C respectively. A synthetic three-strain vaccine against foot-and-mouth disease seems to be within reach.

Given that one can in principle complete the technological chain from nucleic acid sequence to synthetic-peptide vaccine, the next step is to explore certain aspects of vaccine design in more detail. Current research is aimed at finding additional and more sophisticated ways to pinpoint the regions of viral proteins that are most vulnerable to immunological attack and also ways to confer immunity of long duration.

There are essentially two kinds of region in viral proteins. In one kind of region variation is allowed; indeed, it is essential if the virus is to confound the host's immune system. A vaccine that gives rise to antibodies against such a region (HA1 of influenza or VP1 of foot-and-mouth disease, for example) can be expected to be immunogenic, but it must be tailored to cope with each variant strain. There are other regions in viral proteins that have a constant and essential biological function and whose structure cannot vary. The amino acid sequence of such a region is highly conserved among all strains of the virus. If an essential and conserved region is accessible to antibodies, a vaccine that elicits antibodies against it should be a universal vaccine, one from which the virus cannot escape.

The influenza virus is notorious for its ability to evade the immune system by changing parts of the hemagglutinin on its surface. The changes are in the HA1 chain, and, as shown in Figure 7.8, it was peptides from HA1 that we first tested for immunogenicity in the experiment I described above. The hemagglutinin has at least two other and unvarying functions, however. It forms a socket that binds to sialic acid, a sugar on the surface of cells, thereby initiating the infective process. It also causes the surface membranes of infected cells to fuse together, increasing viral infectivity. Evidence from a number of studies by Purnell W. Choppin of Rockefeller University and his colleagues and Michael Waterfield of the Imperial Cancer Research Fund suggests that a conserved region at the beginning of the HA2 chain is at least partly responsible for the fusion.

Normally the immune system does not "see" this region; antibodies to it are usually not made in the course of natural infection. If such antibodies were made (if the region were not only highly conserved and biologically essential but also naturally immunogenic), every human being and other animal host would long since have become immune to the influenza virus; there would be no influenza. We decided to see whether a synthetic peptide from the region might elicit antibodies that would neutralize more than one strain of the virus.

Stephen Alexander, Hannah Alexander and Nicola Green synthesized several peptides from the beginning of the HA2 molecule; the amino acid sequence they chose was that of influenza type A, subtype H_3. Rabbit antiserums against these peptides effectively neutralized the A, H_3 virus when they were tested in a tissue-culture system, showing that even if this region of the HA2 molecule is not normally immunogenic, it is accessible to specific antipeptide antibodies. Moreover, the same antiserums neutralized viruses of a different subtype and even a different major type (influenza B). In contrast, antibodies elicited against the intact H_3 subtype of the virus did not neutralize other subtypes. Nor, of course, are individuals immunized by the injection of one influenza subtype thereby immunized against infection by a different subtype. Much more study of the anti-HA2 antibodies is needed, but these first results suggest that much may be expected of vaccines designed to attack a conserved region having an important biological function.

One way to design a vaccine, then, may be to choose for synthesis a region of a protein that can be expected, on theoretical grounds, to serve as an

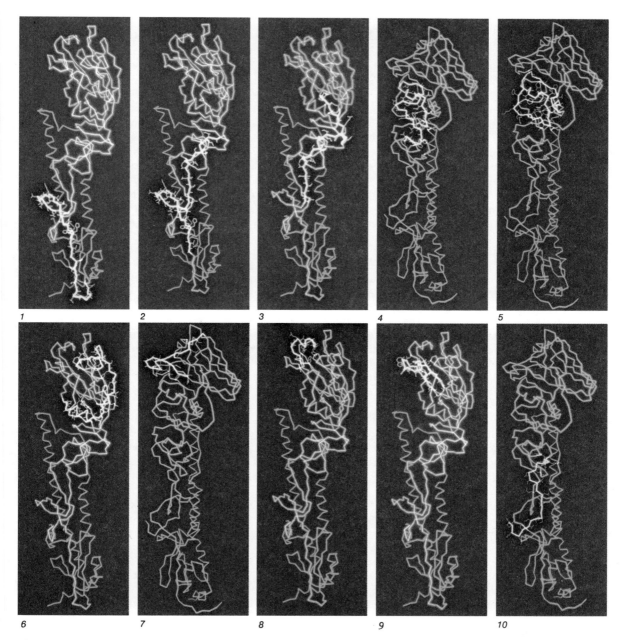

Figure 7.8 SERIES OF PEPTIDES accounting for some 75 percent of the *HA*1 chain was synthesized and each peptide was tested for its ability to elicit antibodies reacting with the peptide, with the hemagglutinin molecule as a whole and with the influenza virus particle. Ten of the 20 peptides tested are shown in yellow in these displays, with their side chains in orange, the remainder of the *HA*1 chain in light blue and the *HA*2 chain in dark blue; in each case the hemagglutinin monomer has been rotated to show the peptide in question to best advantage. When injected into rabbits, most of the peptides elicited antibodies that reacted with the virus, supporting the concept of synthetic-peptide vaccines.

antigenic determinant. There is another way to proceed. One can try to mimic antigenic determinants that have already been shown to be important by seroepidemiologic studies, in which closely related viruses are classified on the basis of the antibodies they elicit. Such studies reveal the existence of different types and subtypes of a virus, such as those I have alluded to in discussing foot-and-mouth disease and influenza.

The types are defined by long-term studies in which viruses responsible for a disease are collected from various areas and at different times. Antibodies taken from patients are tested against the panel of viruses; different antibodies react with different strains of the virus because they "see" different antigenic determinants. By testing many antibodies against a panel of viruses serologists can describe a given virus type in terms of its pattern of determinants and can learn which determinants have been operative in a particular individual or epidemic. Until recently, however, the determinants were abstract "markers" designated by letters or numbers; they were not understood in molecular terms. It was therefore not at all clear that the vast amount of accumulated seroepidemiologic data could help in the design of vaccines. Synthetic peptides might not mimic the structures responsible for serologic markers, for example, if those structures were discontinuous in nature. We decided to try to design a vaccine against the liver disease hepatitis B by synthesizing peptides that would be the molecular equivalent of abstract serologic determinants that have been shown to be important.

The viral component that appears to be the major target of neutralizing antibody, the hepatitis-B surface antigen, is a protein on the envelope of the virus particle. Serologic studies show that the several strains of the hepatitis-B virus have in common one determinant, which is designated a. Each strain also has two other determinants: either d or y and either w or r. That means there are four possible types of the virus: adw, ayw, adr and ayr. Working with John L. Gerin of the Georgetown University School of Medicine and Robert H. Purcell of the National Institute of Allergy and Infectious Diseases, we wanted to synthesize peptides that would specifically elicit antibodies against the d and the y determinants. The hepatitis-B surface antigen, however, is a chain of 226 amino acids. We needed a guide to where to begin. Analysis of the antigen's amino acid sequence in three strains of the virus by

several investigators had shown that there are substantial differences among the strains in only one region of the protein, between amino acids 110 and 140. Any difference in determinants must originate with differences in amino acid sequences, and so that region was clearly the place to seek our peptides.

Following one of the three available amino acid sequences, we synthesized several peptides spanning the region and made antibody to each of them. One 13–amino acid peptide (positions 125 to 137) elicited antibody that reacted only with viruses bearing the y determinants. This meant that the y determinant and its alternative, the d determinant, must lie within the 13–amino acid peptide. Having synthesized y, we should be able to synthesize d by following a different one of the other known sequences for that region. The sequence we chose next differs from the first one at just three positions: two threonines and a tyrosine are replaced respectively by proline, asparagine and phenylalanine. Antibody to the new peptide reacted only with viruses bearing the d determinant.

Perhaps the switch from y to d is brought about by fewer than three amino acid substitutions. By synthesizing peptides in which only one of the three positions is changed at a time we should soon learn whether one, two or all three of the substitutions are required. So far the experiment has taught us two things. One is that very subtle changes in the amino acid composition of a protein can define different strains of a virus. The other is that synthetic peptides can mimic the distinctions revealed by serologic studies; in designing synthetic vaccines one will be able to take advantage of serologic evidence and thereby, for example, attempt to cope with a current epidemic occasioned by a mutant strain.

Before synthetic vaccines can become an alternative to conventional ones ways must be found to increase the magnitude and duration of the immunity they confer. An advantage of attenuated viruses, as I have mentioned, is that they keep proliferating and thus present ever more antigen to the immune system, thereby increasing the antibody level. A synthetic peptide, like a killed virus, does not replicate, and so substances called adjuvants must be added to the vaccine to increase the level and duration of immunity.

One of the most powerful of these, Freund's adjuvant, is an emulsion of mineral oil and water mixed with killed bacteria (mycobacteria, a class that includes the agent of tuberculosis). Just how it works is not known, but it probably does two things. The emulsion retains antigen trapped in it, forming a depot from which antigen is released slowly, simulating the sustained presentation of antigen by a replicating virus. Meanwhile the killed bacteria attract to the depot various cells that have roles in the immune response. To attract such cells is also to serve as an irritant, however, causing soreness at the site of injection and even the formation of an abscess. Powerful adjuvants such as Freund's may not be administered to human beings; instead, alum, or aluminum hydroxide, is commonly included with a killed-virus vaccine. The antigen is adsorbed onto the aluminum hydroxide particles and is released slowly after injection. In some cases, it appears, alum will serve well enough with synthetic vaccines, but most such vaccines will require something better. Much effort is currently aimed at the development of safe and effective adjuvants.

Some hopeful results in this direction have been reported by François Audibert and Louis Chedid of the Pasteur Institute and Ruth Arnon and Michael Sela of the Weizmann Institute of Science, who recently elicited antibodies conferring passive immunity against the diphtheria toxin. They synthesized three peptides corresponding to regions of the toxin molecule. Before injection a synthetic peptide must be coupled to a carrier molecule. (In all our experiments the carrier was keyhole-limpet hemocyanin, a respiratory pigment of a mollusk, which is often used for this purpose.) The Pasteur-Weizmann group devised a carrier-adjuvant combination. They coupled their diphtheria-toxin peptides to a carrier that had been linked to a simple derivative of the cell membrane of mycobacteria; the membrane derivative apparently serves as an adjuvant, significantly increasing the immunogenicity of the peptides.

As I mentioned at the beginning of this article, antipeptide antibodies should have important applications as investigative tools. One application arises from advances in nucleic acid technology. Because of the precision of recombinant-DNA techniques and the remarkable speed of the new methods for determining the sequence of a nucleic acid, it is often the case that one has the complete sequence of a gene before the protein it encodes is known; one has a gene in search of a protein. From the DNA or RNA sequence one can now predict an amino acid sequence and select a small region of it for synthesis. Antibodies elicited by the peptide

serve as a probe for finding the protein. By this means, for example, the proteins encoded by some oncogenes, the tumor-inducing genes of certain viruses, have been identified and tracked to particular sites in cells.

The distinguishing feature of antipeptide antibodies is of course their predetermined specificity. They are antibodies not to a protein but to a particular part of the protein that is known to the experimenter. Once they have been manufactured by the immune system of a laboratory animal they can easily be purified by a single passage through an immunoadsorbent column. Then they can be used to explore in detail the structure of a protein and to correlate the structure with function. For example, antibodies to a particular part of a protein will bind to that part and inhibit its function, and so tests with a battery of peptides should make it possible to define the active site of a protein or various sites that are active in different functions. Again, many peptide hormones originate in a long protein chain that is subsequently cleaved by an enzyme into smaller pieces, each one a hormone with a particular activity. Antibodies to peptides serve to sort out the cleaved pieces and correlate each with its activity.

Finally, antibodies of predetermined specificity can reveal just which part of a gene is being expressed to make a protein at a particular time. Mammalian genes are split into a number of the coding regions called exons. In the case of certain variable proteins different exons are expressed at different times. Successive forms of antibody molecules are synthesized, for example, in the course of the immune response. Now one can synthesize the peptide encoded by each exon, make antibody to it and learn which exon is being expressed at a particular stage of the immune response.

POSTSCRIPT

Biotechnology promises to revolutionize the control of infectious disease. New drugs, new diagnostic procedures and new vaccines can all be anticipated to result from the new field of biotechnology. Some approaches to the production of completely synthetic vaccines have been described. Vaccines, the most ancient of medical interventions, can now be produced by the most modern techniques of biotechnology.

There are a number of problems with conventional vaccines that synthetic vaccines might overcome. Among these problems, safety is perhaps the most important. Conventional vaccines are made either by attenuating or killing the infectious agent, but there is always the possibility that an attenuated agent might revert to the virulent form and cause disease. With killed agents, the procedure for killing may not always be properly done, so that infectious material remains intact in the vaccine. A synthetic vaccine would not have a safety problem because at no time is the infectious agent itself involved in its production.

Vaccines work because they bring about the production of antibodies that neutralize infectious agents. With a virus, the antibody combines with protein subunits (capsids) on the surface of the virus particle. The virus proteins that elicit antibody formation are thus antigens. Each antigenic protein of the virus has a number of potential sites at which an antibody can combine. Each of these sites is called an antigenic determinant, which may be formed from a continuous sequence of amino acids or may consist of amino acids from different parts of the protein molecule that are brought together as a result of the folding of the protein. In order for an appropriate synthetic vaccine to be made, it is nec-

essary to know exactly which amino acids the antibody combines with. Thus, it is important to know the configuration of the virus protein. Computer modeling techniques have made it possible to visualize the manner by which the amino acids of the virus proteins are arranged. The success of the synthetic vaccine program is thus linked to the availability of sophisticated high-speed computing.

It is important to emphasize that a synthetic peptide by itself will not be an effective vaccine. This is because small peptides are not very effective in eliciting antibody formation. It is only when the synthetic peptide is linked to a larger carrier molecule that it can be used as a successful vaccine. Thus, delivery of the vaccine is also an important research activity.

Although the production of synthetic vaccines holds great promise, much research will be needed before such vaccines replace the currently available conventional vaccines. Also, continued research to develop new conventional vaccines will still be needed, since the development of synthetic vaccines requires detailed knowledge of the structures of the infectious agents, knowledge that is often not readily available.

PROTOZOAL DISEASES OUT OF AFRICA

. . .

Introduction to Section III

Although the infectious diseases that have been the most widespread in the Western world have been caused by bacteria or viruses, in Africa some of the most important diseases are caused by a completely different group of microorganisms, the protozoa. The protozoa are one-celled animals that cause diseases primarily of the blood, although the parasites sometimes invade the nervous system or body organs. Because protozoa are animals, their structure and metabolism resemble more closely those of humans than do the bacteria. This has made it difficult to discover specific therapeutic drugs, because often a drug that will target a protozoan will also be toxic to human cells.

Another reason for the difficulty of controlling these diseases is that Africa itself is a "difficult" continent. Beginning with the cruel and barbarous exploitation of Africa by Europeans since the 15th century, Africa has always been treated as a source of European wealth rather than as the home of millions of human beings. Europeans colonized Africa most extensively beginning in the late 19th century, and the continent was divided up between the British, Portuguese, French and Germans. The Boer War of 1899–1902 resulted in British dominance over South Africa. After World War I, the German colonies were appropriated and transferred to the Allied Powers under the League of Nations. It was only after World War II that a rise in nationalism occurred in Africa, resulting eventually in independence for virtually all the African countries. However, the European legacies remained, for the modern countries of Africa follow boundaries established by the European colonizers. Racial and religious differences, tribal groupings and difficult climatic regimes have made much of Africa a major medical challenge. It is not accidental that the last stand of smallpox was in the African country of Ethiopia (see Chapter 5, "The Eradication of Smallpox").

If the protozoan diseases of Africa also were of widespread occurrence in the West, there would be vast research establishments devoted to their study and eradication. As it is, only a few dedicated individuals carry on the research essential for an understanding of these major diseases. Profit-making pharmaceutical companies focus their research on diseases for which a viable market exists, and research funding of Western governments is devoted primarily to similar diseases. Often, it is only the military establishment that supports research on African diseases, because the military must always anticipate sending soldiers to remote parts of the world.

In this section the two most important protozoal diseases of Africa are discussed: malaria and trypanosomiasis (African sleeping sickness). Although malaria is most commonly identified with Africa, it occurs throughout the world in the tropical and subtropical regions. African sleeping sickness is restricted to central Africa, but its widespread distribution and difficulty of control have made it an important disease. Trypanosomiasis has also proved to be of great interest as a model research system for studying the genetics of parasitism, and the research presented here opens up new vistas. For both malaria and trypanosomiasis, recombinant DNA techniques have made possible quite sophisticated research studies.

The Biochemistry of Resistance to Malaria

Genes for two lethal diseases, sickle-cell anemia and thalassemia, are favored by evolution because they protect against malaria. Now the mechanisms of that protection can be studied in the laboratory.

· · ·

Milton J. Friedman and William Trager
March, 1981

Evolution results from natural selection, operating over a range of genetic diversity that arises from the mutation and recombination of genes. Variant genes that confer some selective advantage tend to increase in frequency, whereas deleterious variants tend to be eliminated. In human populations there are very few clear examples of selection for or against specific genes in response to specific forces. The best examples are inherited diseases. Selection acts against the genes that cause such diseases, and it acts most strongly against the severest conditions.

That being the case, lethal genetic diseases should be very rare. Yet certain inherited disorders of the red blood cells, notably sickle-cell anemia and thalassemia, are observed in some populations at surprisingly high frequencies. Does that argue against natural selection? On the contrary, the sickle-cell and thalassemia genes demonstrate the force of selection in evolution. The same variant genes that cause lethal blood-cell disease in homozygous individuals (who inherit two of the abnormal genes, one from each parent) protect heterozygous individuals (who inherit one abnormal gene and one normal gene) against the lethal effects of malaria, the agent of which is a parasite that infects red blood cells.

That protection maintains the high frequencies of these otherwise deleterious genes.

The strength of malaria as a selective force derives from the powerful effect of the parasitic disease on the health and reproductive capacity of human populations. Malaria has been a major cause of death throughout history. In Africa today malaria is endemic: it does not sweep through a population as an epidemic but rather is a constant affliction contributing to early-childhood mortality rates as high as 50 percent. It kills about 10 percent of its victims directly and contributes to the death of others by decreasing the immune system's ability to fight other infections. Because of malaria a significant number of children do not live to reproduce. Any genetic mutation that provides resistance to malaria must therefore have a high selective advantage.

It was the coincidence of the geographic range of sickle-cell disease with the range of malaria that first drew attention to the possibility that the sickle-cell gene might confer such resistance (see Figure 8.1). Clinical evidence was harder to come by, but in 1954 Anthony C. Allison of the University of Oxford showed that children who were heterozygous for the sickle-cell gene had much less severe cases of the most lethal form of the disease than children who did not carry the gene. Because the parasite that causes malaria could not be maintained in a laboratory culture, however, the resistance could not be demonstrated at the cellular level, nor could its biochemical mechanism be established. Recently we have exploited a newly developed culture system to learn how the sickle-cell gene and some other variant genes that alter red-cell function confer resistance to malaria.

The red blood cell, where the malaria parasite encounters the altered cellular functions governed by these variant genes, is largely filled with hemoglobin: the protein that takes on oxygen in the lungs and carries it to the tissues. The other proteins of the red-cell cytoplasm are metabolic enzymes. (The biochemical processes in the red blood cell are shown in Figure 8.2.) Some of them catalyze glycolysis, whereby glucose is broken down step by step

to form lactate, in the process synthesizing adenosine triphosphate (ATP). Others catalyze what is called the hexose monophosphate shunt, which maintains the coenzymes nicotinamide adenine dinucleotide phosphate (NADP) and glutathione in their reduced form. ATP is the all-purpose cellular energy carrier; reduced NADP (NADPH) and reduced glutathione are needed to prevent and repair oxidative damage. The cell membrane bounds the cell and controls its shape and deformability. It also controls the movement of ions into the cell and out of it; in particular it maintains—at the expense of ATP—a high-potassium interior against a tendency toward equilibrium with the low-potassium outside environment. On the outside of the membrane glycoproteins and glycolipids present a unique recognizable surface to the environment.

It is at this surface that the malaria parasite first interacts with the cell. The parasite is a small unicellular protozoon of the genus *Plasmodium*, four spe-

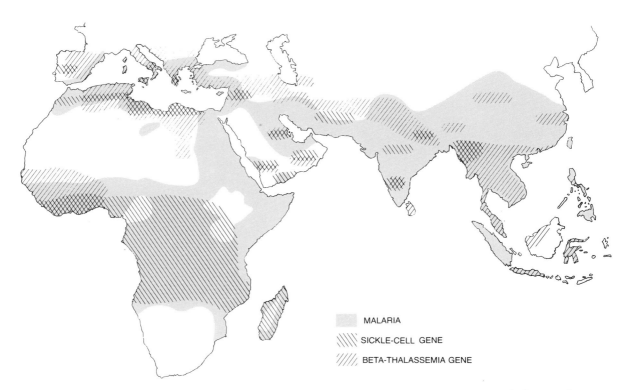

MALARIA

SICKLE-CELL GENE

BETA-THALASSEMIA GENE

Figure 8.1 DISTRIBUTIONS of the sickle-cell gene and of the beta-thalassemia gene lie within the area where falciparum malaria was prevalent before 1930 (*color*). This geographic coincidence provided the first suggestion that re- **sistance to malaria might be the evolutionary advantage that was tending to maintain the genes responsible for lethal blood diseases at high frequencies in certain human populations.**

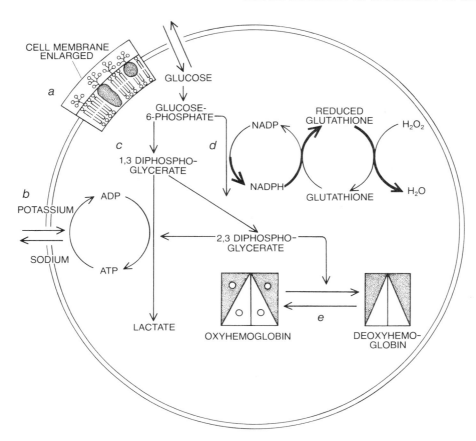

Figure 8.2 RED BLOOD CELL. Glycolipids and glycoproteins on the surface (*a*) determine the cell's interactions with its environment and with the malaria parasite. Proteins in the membrane control the transport of potassium and sodium (*b*). This process requires energy, which is provided by ATP generated through gycolysis, whereby glucose is broken down to form lactate (*c*). The hexose monophosphate shunt (*d*) produces reduced NADP and reduced glutathione. The cytoplasm is largely filled with hemoglobin (*e*), which binds oxygen in the lung and delivers it to the tissues, in the process undergoing structural changes that are to some extent controlled by diphosphoglycerate.

cies of which cause malaria in humans; the most lethal disease, responsible for a million deaths every year among African children, is caused by *Plasmodium falciparum*. A specialized form of the parasite is injected into the bloodstream by an *Anopheles* mosquito, migrates to the liver and there develops and divides to produce merozoites, the form that infects red cells. The merozoites reenter the bloodstream and recognize and bind to the red-cell membrane (see Figure 8.3). A mechanism, as yet poorly understood, is activated that causes the merozoite to push in the cell membrane, which closes around it. Enclosed in a vacuole, the parasite grows, digesting hemoglobin to acquire the amino acids to make its own proteins and, we believe, utilizing red-cell glucose, ATP and reduced coenzymes in its metabolism. After a period of growth the parasite's nucleus divides several times, and then membranes enclose each nucleus and its surrounding cytoplasm. In this manner from 12 to 24 new merozoites are formed, which burst out of the cell and invade other cells.

The characteristic periodic fever of malaria results from the synchronous release of merozoites, and of toxins produced by the parasite, throughout the body. In the case of *P. falciparum* this release takes place every 48 hours, the period of the parasite's

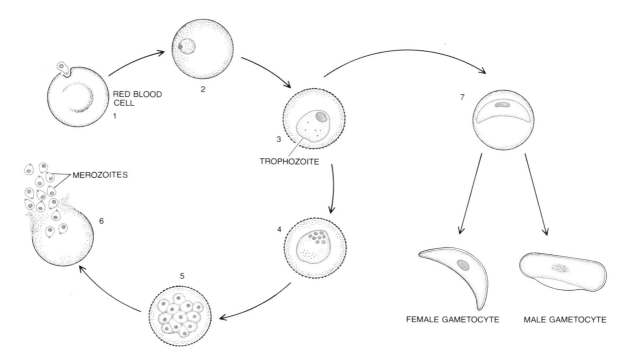

Figure 8.3 LIFE CYCLE of *P. falciparum* in the red cell begins with the invasion of the cell by a merozoite (*1*). The parasite engulfs a droplet of cytoplasm, so that in section it looks like a thin ring (*2*). The ring grows and fills in to become a trophozoite (*3*); knoblike structures develop on the cell surface and attach the cell to the blood-vessel wall. There the parasite's nucleus divides repeatedly (*4*); each daughter nucleus acquires a bit of cytoplasm (*5*), and the parasite divides into from 12 to 24 merozoites, which burst the cell and begin a new cycle (*6*). Some trophozoites develop (*7*) into male and female gametocytes, which are ingested by mosquitoes to initiate the sexual phase of the cycle.

developmental cycle in the red cell. The fever and the debilitation that accompany it are the major symptoms of malaria. In falciparum malaria, however, there is a more lethal effect. The infected red cell develops knobs on its surface that attach the cell to the walls of capillaries, where it lodges until the parasite is mature. When a large number of cells are thus sequestered in a vital organ such as the brain, death can result. The clearest indication of the protective effect of the sickle-cell gene is that very few carriers of the gene die from the cerebral complications of falciparum malaria.

Linus Pauling and his colleagues defined a molecular disease for the first time when they demonstrated that in sickle-cell anemia the hemoglobin molecule is altered, and that people with sickle-cell disease have only the altered molecule, hemoglobin *S*, in their red cells, whereas some members of their families have about half hemoglobin *S* and half normal hemoglobin *A*. Family studies published at about the same time confirmed Pauling's findings, showing that the inheritance pattern of sickle-cell anemia could be ascribed to a single gene, with the disease appearing only in family members who are homozygous for that gene (see Figure 8.4).

Adult hemoglobin is made up of two alpha chains and two beta chains, and Vernon M. Ingram of the University of Cambridge soon showed that in hemoglobin *S* only the beta chain is abnormal. The abnormality involves only one of the amino acids constituting the chain: a valine is substituted for a glutamic acid. Sickle-cell homozygotes (designated *SS*) have only hemoglobin *S* because they carry two of the mutant beta-chain genes. Heterozygotes (*AS*), who are said to have sickle-cell "trait," carry only one mutant beta-chain gene, and about 40 percent of their hemoglobin is hemoglobin *S*. If two people with sickle-cell trait have four children, the proba-

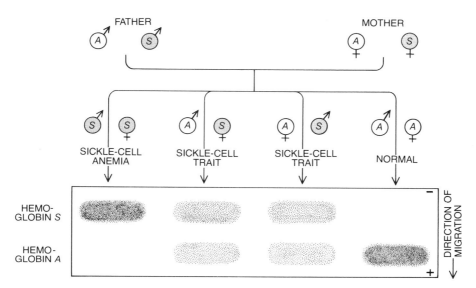

Figure 8.4 INHERITANCE of genes for abnormal hemoglobin S is diagrammed for parents who are heterozygous for the abnormal gene. One child is homozygous (*SS*) for the gene, and has sickle-cell anemia. Two children inherit one gene for hemoglobin *S* and one for normal hemoglobin *A*; they are heterozygous (*AS*) and have sickle-cell "trait." One child is normal (*AA*). Hemoglobin samples placed on cellulose acetate are subjected to an electric current (*bottom*). Hemoglobin *S* differs from hemoglobin *A* in only one amino acid, which lacks a negative charge, and so hemoglobin *S* migrates toward the positive pole less rapidly than hemoglobin *A*.

bility is, in accordance with Mendelian principles, that one child will have sickle-cell disease, one will be normal and two will have sickle-cell trait.

The symptoms of sickle-cell disease appear when the *SS* red blood cells lose oxygen as they circulate through the tissues. When hemoglobin *S* is dexoygenated, it tends to aggregate in long, thin fibers (see Figure 8.5). The fibers distort the normally disk-shaped cells into angular forms, including the characteristic crescent shape. In a sickle-cell crisis some sickled cells block the local circulation of blood and impede the delivery of oxygen. As the oxygen level drops, more red cells sickle and the area of impaired circulation spreads, causing extensive tissue death. In the absence of advanced medical treatment the survival of hemoglobin-*S* homozygotes is very low. People with sickle-cell trait do not ordinarily suffer from the disease, however. Their *AS* red cells have enough normal hemoglobin so that they sickle only under extreme conditions, such as at high altitudes.

Since *Plasmodium falciparum* is an obligate parasite, it cannot be cultured away from living cells, and for many years research on this parasite has been thwarted. It has now been possible to define the conditions that make it possible to maintain *P. falciparum* in a continuous culture of human red blood cells in an artificial bloodlike medium (see Figure 8.6). The culture system is being exploited by some workers to develop experimental vaccines containing material from various stages of the parasite's life cycle, which are being tested in animals. Other investigators are trying to purify and analyze the biochemical agents that have particular effects in the course of an infection. The system has also made it possible for us to study in detail the interactions of the malaria parasite and variant host red cells.

To learn how sickle-cell hemoglobin protects a heterozygote carrier against malaria we cultured the malaria parasite in red blood cells taken from normal donors, from individuals with sickle-cell trait and from patients with sickle-cell anemia. (The stages in the culture procedure are shown in Figure 8.7). We did so under our standard culture conditions, in an atmosphere with an oxygen concentration of 17 percent, which created an oxygen tension in the culture medium similar to that in the lungs; the hemoglobin was fully oxygenated and the variant cells did not sickle. Under these conditions the parasites grew equally well in all three kinds of

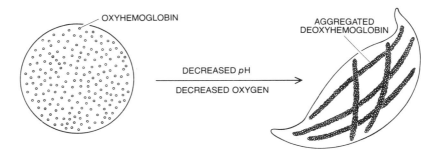

Figure 8.5 HEMOGLOBIN S in its oxygenated state (*left*) is dispersed through the red cell, which has a normal disk shape. Unlike normal hemoglobin A, however, hemoglobin S tends to aggregate when it becomes deoxygenated in the tissues, forming needlelike quasi-crystalline structures that distort the cell into a rigid, jagged shape (*right*). Sickled cells may block capillaries, decreasing blood flow, reducing the oxygen level and thus promoting the sickling of more cells.

cells. This showed that there is no major alteration of red-cell metabolism in the variant cells, and that hemoglobin S, like hemoglobin A, can be digested by the plasmodium.

To test the effect of sickling on parasite growth we added a small number of infected normal cells to cultures of SS and AS cells in a 17 percent oxygen atmosphere. During the next 48 hours, the period of one growth cycle, all the parasites left their normal host cells and invaded the variant cells. When we

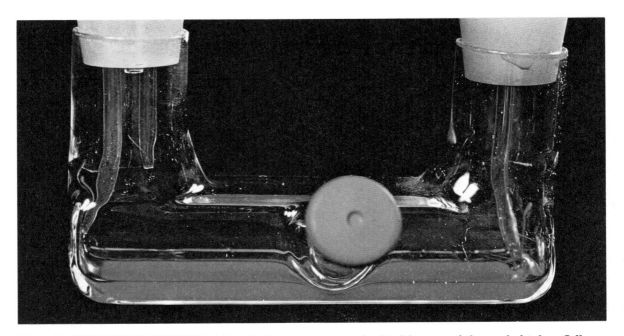

Figure 8.6 CONTINUOUS CULTURE of the malaria parasite *Plasmodium falciparum* can be maintained in this apparatus. The parasites are grown in a thin layer of human red blood cells that coats the bottom of the horizontal tube and is covered with a nutritional medium. The oxygen content of the medium and other experimental conditions are manipulated by way of the vertical tubes. Cells are removed for microscopic analysis through the short tube at the front center. Until conditions for culturing the parasite were established in 1976, research on falciparum malaria, the most lethal form of the disease, had to be done with the blood of human volunteers or primate hosts.

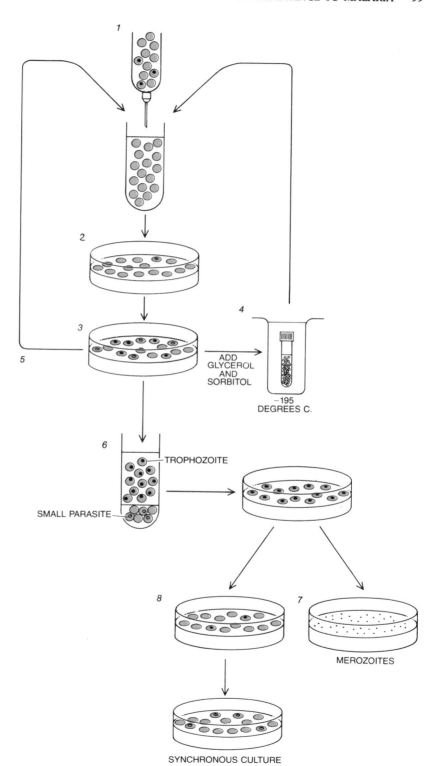

Figure 8.7 *P. FALCIPARUM* CUL-TURE is begun by inoculating fresh human red cells with para-sitized cells from a patient or from a stock culture (*1*). The cells are grown at body temperature as a thin layer covered by a nutrient medium (*2*). After three or four days the cells contain a mixture of small and large parasites (*3*), which can be frozen for future use (*4*), inoculated into new cultures (*5*) or incubated in a gelatin solu-tion to separate trophozoites (*6*); these large parasites can be grown alone to produce merozoites for further study (*7*) or can be mixed with fresh cells to produce a syn-chronous culture of parasites (*8*).

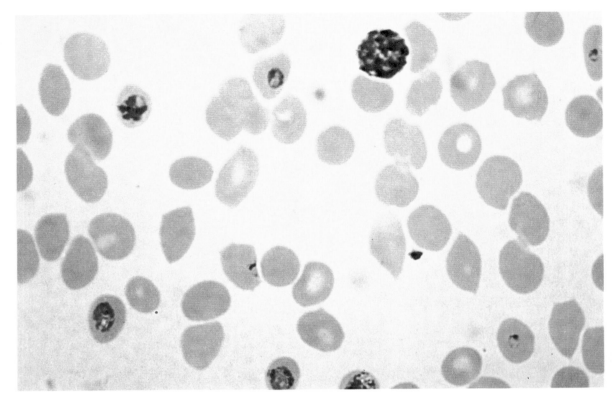

Figure 8.8 FATE OF MALARIA PARASITES is monitored in smears of the cultured cells on microscope slides. The stain (Giemsa's) colors the cell nuclei of the parasites dark purple and the parasite cytoplasm blue. The rate of multi-plication is measured by counting the number of parasites per 100 red cells. This smear shows the parasites at various stages of their life cycle (see Figure 8.3).

lowered the oxygen concentration to 3 percent, the SS cells sickled, as did some of the AS cells. A microscopic method (Figure 8.8) was used to monitor the parasites daily. After one day in low oxygen almost no parasites were visible in the SS-cell cultures; they had lysed, or disintegrated, and so had their host cells (see Figure 8.9). In the AS-cell cultures, on the other hand, it was only on the second day that the number of live parasites decreased significantly. And rather than disintegrating, the killed parasites were still visible as shriveled masses in the cells. They looked to us like parasites that had starved, perhaps as the result of some kind of metabolic inhibition that was an indirect result of sickling.

If that was the case, preventing sickling should protect the parasites. We treated AS cells with cyanate, which increases the affinity of hemoglobin S for oxygen, making it less likely to aggregate at a given

oxygen tension. After cyanate treatment and washing, the AS cells remained competent as hosts for P. falciparum, but now they did not sickle as readily. When such cells were infected and then cultured in 3 percent oxygen, the parasites survived. The inhibition we had seen in untreated cells must therefore have been due to the sickling of the cells, not simply to low oxygen. By what mechanism might sickling inhibit parasite growth?

One of the things that happen when a red cell containing hemoglobin S sickles is that the cell membrane becomes more permeable to potassium, which leaks out; in the low-oxygen condition the potassium level in our AS host cells was decreased (see Figure 8.10). It had earlier been shown that parasites maintained outside red cells require a high-potassium environment, and so we hypothesized that the loss of potassium on sickling might

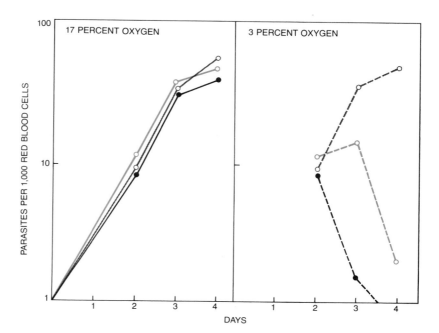

Figure 8.9 MULTIPLICATION OF P. FALCIPARUM is about the same in normal cells (*open circles*), AS cells (*color*) and SS cells (*black*) as long as the cells are in 17 percent oxygen (*left*). If after two days the oxygen level is lowered to 3 percent, however, only parasites in normal cells keep growing (*right*). The parasites in the SS cells die in a day, those in the AS cells in two days.

have inhibited parasite metabolism. To test the idea we again incubated infected AS cells in 3 percent oxygen, but in a medium with an elevated potassium content. The cells sickled as usual in low oxygen, but now the cellular potassium level stayed high—and the parasites survived. Preventing the loss of potassium, in other words, prevented the inhibition of parasite growth in sickled AS cells. (Under the same conditions plasmodia in sickled SS cells were not protected; they died by lysis. Electron micrographs showed why. After six hours of deoxygenation needlelike bundles of aggregated hemoglobin S could be seen penetrating some of the plasmodia; the membranes of other parasites had been disrupted, and they were partially lysed. In other words, in the SS cells the parasites were killed not by metabolic inhibition but by actual physical disruption.)

The sequence of events in AS cells, then, seemed to be as follows: Sickling lowered the potassium level, and the low potassium level killed the parasites. This finding could not, however, fully explain the heterozygote's resistance to malaria. Because an uninfected AS cell has less hemoglobin S than an SS cell, it does not normally sickle in nature; it circulates through regions of low oxygen tension too

quickly for sickling to take place. The progress of a parasitized cell, however, is impeded by the knobs on its surface, and the cell remains in a low-oxygen environment for many hours. Even so, fewer than 5 percent of the cells would sickle were it not for still another effect of infection.

Lucio Luzzatto and his colleagues at the Istituto Internazionale di Genetica e Biofisica in Naples have shown that infected cells sickle much faster than uninfected ones. Why? We found that the intracellular environment of an infected cell is more acidic (.4 pH units lower) than that of an uninfected cell, so that the rate of sickling is significantly increased. We calculate, moreover, that the lower pH level of parasitized cells also increases the extent of sickling—up to about 40 percent.

Taken all together these observations suggest the following mechanism of protection against malaria in sickle-cell heterozygotes. The parasite in an infected AS cell develops normally until the cell is sequestered in the tissues. Then, given the low-oxygen environment and the low intracellular pH, the host cell sickles (see Figure 8.11). The potassium level drops and the parasite dies. Such a process can protect against malaria even if not all the parasites are affected, because even a reduction in the rate of multiplication of the plasmodium can give the im-

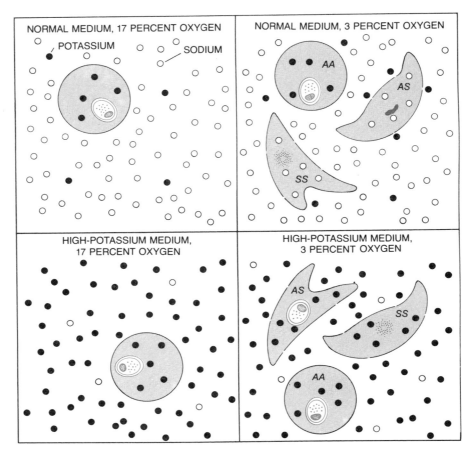

Figure 8.10 POTASSIUM LOSS is shown to be the cause of parasite death in *AS* cells. In 17 percent oxygen (*left*) the cell membrane remains intact and the potassium level is adequately maintained in either a normal physiological (low potassium) medium (*top*) or in elevated potassium (*bottom*). In a low-oxygen, low-potassium medium (*top right*) *AS* and *SS* cells sickle; their membranes are disrupted, they lose potassium and their parasites shrivel up (*AS*) or disappear (*SS*). Incubation in a high-potassium medium (*bottom right*) protects parasites in *AS* cells in spite of sickling and membrane disruption, but it does not protect parasites in *SS* cells.

mune system the time it needs to mount a protective response of its own. (There is an alternative hypothesis. Infected cells might, for some reason we have not discerned, sickle while circulating rather than while being sequestered, and then they might be eliminated by the filtering action of the spleen. The first hypothesis is supported, however, by evidence that heterozygotes are not protected against types of malaria in which infected cells do not develop knobs and are not sequestered in the tissues.)

In addition to sickle-cell disease and sickle-cell trait there are other inherited disorders of the red blood cells whose geographic incidence has been correlated with that of malaria, implying that the genes responsible for those disorders too may confer some resistance. Among those disorders are the thalassemias, which involve a deficiency in the manufacture of one or another hemoglobin chain. Beta thalassemia, for example, is a deficiency in beta-chain synthesis. Homozygous beta thalassemia, known as Cooley's anemia, is a severe disease in which little normal adult hemoglobin, if any, is synthesized; blood transfusion is usually the only means by which a patient's life can be prolonged. Yet throughout many malarial regions, and in particular around the rim of the Mediterranean, about 1

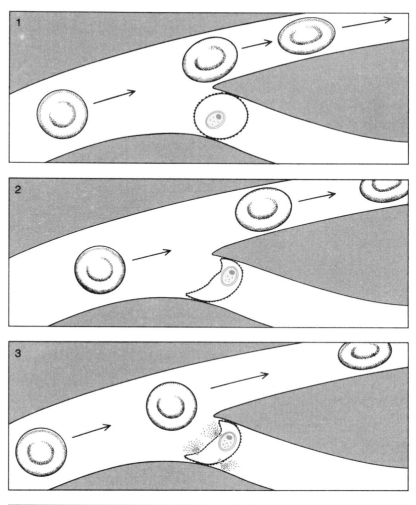

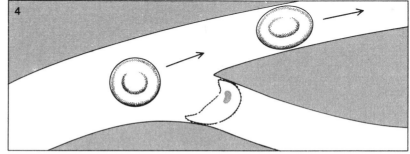

Figure 8.11 CHAIN OF EVENTS depicted here may protect *AS* heterozygotes against malaria. A parasite-infected cell is characterized by knobs on its surface and by a low intracellular *p*H. An uninfected *AS* cell will pass through a short period of low oxygenation in a capillary without sickling (*1*); an infected cell, on the other hand, will be sequestered long enough so that the low oxygen level and the low *p*H cause it to sickle (*2*). Sickling causes the cell membrane to leak potassium (*3*). Deprived of potassium, the parasite dies (*4*). The death of some fraction of the infecting parasites may give the heterozygote's body time to develop its own immune response.

percent of all children born are homozygous for the beta-thalassemia gene and have Cooley's anemia; heterozygotes do not have the disease. Resistance to malaria has not been convincingly demonstrated for beta-thalassemia heterozygotes, but there is a very suggestive geographic correlation between the frequency of the gene and a regional history of malaria. To cite just one example, the gene frequency is much higher in the valleys of Sardinia, where malaria was for a long time endemic, than it is in the mountains, where malaria was rarer.

We set out to demonstrate a resistance effect in our culture system. We knew that one characteristic of any thalassemic cell is abnormal sensitivity of the cell membrane to damage by oxidation. When a molecule is oxidized, electrons are removed that would ordinarily have a role in the formation of chemical bonds. When lipid (fat) molecules, which are major constituents of the membrane, are oxidized, they fragment and disrupt the integrity of the membrane. The agents of oxidation in cells have not all been identified, but it is known that one such agent is hydrogen peroxide.

The malaria parasite generates hydrogen peroxide in its host cell (as has been demonstrated by N. Etkin and John W. Eaton of the University of Minnesota Medical School). Peroxides give rise in any cell to oxidative stress, challenging the cell's ability to preserve its integrity. In the more sensitive thalassemic red cell hydrogen peroxide might actually bring about damage to the membrane. We confirmed the likelihood of this effect by finding that parasites in heterozygous beta-thalassemia cells were more sensitive than parasites in normal cells to three experimental conditions. One condition was a high-oxygen environment (an oxygen concentration of from 25 to 30 percent). Another was the presence of certain chemicals that catalyze oxidation reactions. The third was the absence from the culture medium of one normal constituent: reduced glutathione, which is an intermediate in the metabolic pathway that reduces the cellular level of hydrogen peroxide.

Each of these three conditions was calculated to increase the oxidative stress on the cell. Eaton found that in mice infected with malaria oxidative stress and protection against it are finely balanced. Any additional sensitivity in a thalassemic cell, therefore, might well affect the course of the infection. (Although a thalassemic cell has a low hemoglobin content, there is apparently enough hemoglobin to maintain the parasite; the low hemoglobin level alone did not inhibit parasite multiplication in our system.)

We found that vitamin E, which protects cell-membrane lipids against oxidative damage, prevented the death of parasites in thalassemia-trait cells under all conditions. This was supporting evidence for the idea that the membrane of a heterozygous beta-thalassemia cell is damaged by oxidation in the course of malaria infection. As for the mechanism, again potassium appears to be implicated. In a high-potassium medium the parasites in the thalassemia-trait cells developed normally under conditions that led to their death in a medium with a normal potassium concentration.

There were three interesting corollary results of this investigation. One was the reinforcement of a long-suspected link between malaria and an inherited deficiency in the red cell's supply of the enzyme glucose-6-phosphate dehydrogenase (G6PD). This deficiency too is prevalent in malarial regions; field studies have sometimes, but not always, demonstrated a correlation with resistance to malaria. G6PD is the first enzyme in the hexose monophosphate shunt, which regenerates NADPH, a coenzyme that is essential for protection against and repair of oxidative damage. It appeared that red cells deficient in G6PD, like thalassemia-trait cells, might be more sensitive to the hydrogen peroxide generated by the malaria parasite. We found that parasites in G6PD-deficient cells were indeed highly sensitive to stress by oxidants and were protected by antioxidant agents.

A second corollary implication of our results with thalassemic cells had to do with favism: a hemolytic anemia promoted by the ingestion of fava beans, which are consumed throughout the Mediterranean world. The fava bean contains a variety of substances that could increase the red cell's sensitivity to oxidants; some of the substances are related to the oxidation catalysts introduced in some of our experiments. Do those experiments mimic the consumption of fava beans by people with beta-thalassemic or G6PD-deficient red cells? If they do, the results would indicate that eating fava beans (and perhaps other foods as yet not identified) increases the level of protection against malaria in people who are heterozygous for these two red-cell disorders. Such a dietary effect could also explain the inconsistent results of studies of malaria resistance among such heterozygotes.

The third corollary result had to do with infants. During the first few months of life infants are almost completely protected against malaria. Geoffrey Pasvol, R. J. M. Wilson and D. J. Weatherall of the University of Oxford recently showed that fetal hemoglobin (which consists of alpha and gamma chains, persists for a time after birth and is found in some adults' red cells) may contribute to this protection; even adult red cells inhibited the growth of parasites if the cells contained fetal hemoglobin. We have found that malaria parasites in fetal red cells, like those in thalassemic cells, are highly sensitive to oxidative stress. It is not likely that malaria has been a selective force in the evolution of fetal hemoglobin, however. The fetal protein probably evolved under a different selective pressure. It has a higher affinity for oxygen than adult hemoglobin, and so it improves the delivery of oxygen to the developing fetus. The oxidant sensitivity of the fetal red cell and the resulting resistance to malaria are probably side effects of a developmental adaptation.

To sum up, the process of evolution has resulted in the selection of genetically variant red blood cells that function well enough under normal conditions but are susceptible to damage when they are infected by *P. falciparum*—damage that kills the parasite. In other words, these cells are so marginally viable that infection makes them unviable and unable to support the intracellular parasite. The genetic alteration in the case of *AS* cells is a borderline tendency to sickle, which is enhanced by the parasite's presence. The alteration in thalassemia-trait cells is increased sensitivity of the membrane lipids to hydrogen peroxide generated by the parasite. In both cases the end effect is a loss of potassium that inhibits the parasite's metabolism.

The evolutionary career of a gene can be quite complex. When a new random mutation arises, one cannot predict its effect or its potential. One could surely not have predicted that certain genes would cause lethal blood disease in a homozygote and protect the heterozygote against death from malaria. The delicately balanced contest between the selective effect of malaria on the one hand and of sickle-cell disease and beta thalassemia on the other has resulted in a balanced polymorphism: a situation in which a heterozygote advantage coupled with a homozygote disadvantage maintains a variant gene at a low but consistent level in a population.

The mechanisms of life and death are rooted in chemistry and molecular biology. They can be explicated, to some extent, in the laboratory. Their ultimate effects on the human species are decided, however, not in the laboratory or even in the cells of individual human beings but slowly and unpredictably in evolutionary contests waged across continents and over millenniums.

POSTSCRIPT

In terms of the number of humans affected, malaria ranks as the most important of all infectious diseases. Although now confined primarily to tropical and subtropical regions where its mosquito vector flourishes, in earlier years malaria occurred extensively even in temperate regions. Control of malaria was brought about in temperate countries when swamps and wetlands in which mosquitoes breed were drained. During World War II in areas of the world where military activities occurred, the U.S. military inaugurated major malaria control programs. After the war the introduction of the insecticide DDT played a major role in reducing malaria incidence in the tropics, but the mosquito gradually developed resistance to this chemical so that malaria still flourishes in these areas.

The malaria parasite was first seen in the blood in 1880 by the French scientist Charles Laveran, a discovery for which he was awarded the Nobel Prize in 1907. The connection between the malaria parasite and the mosquito was shown by the British physician Ronald Ross near the end of the 19th century. Ross was a medical officer in the British army in India and made extensive studies of the transmission of the malaria parasite by the mosquito. Working in Bombay, Ross allowed human volunteers to be bitten by malaria-containing mosquitoes and later found the malaria parasite in their red blood cells. To permit more careful studies, Ross turned to malaria of birds, a related disease, and was able to demonstrate unequivocally the role of the mosquito. Finally, in 1898, he was able to describe the complete life cycle of the malaria parasite. He returned to England in 1899 and was awarded the Nobel Prize in 1902.

Long before the cause of malaria was determined, the antimalarial properties of the bark of the cinchona tree were known. The active principle, quinine, was isolated early in the 19th century, one of the first chemotherapeutic agents ever developed. At the turn of the 20th century, the chemical structure of quinine had been determined and the drug was synthesized. Soon chemists had produced a vast array of quinine-related drugs, of which the most effective was chloroquin. Although this agent helped to control malaria throughout the world, the malaria parasite has gradually developed resistance to the drug, so that today chemical treatment is much less certain.

Although the life cycle of malaria has been known for a long time, the connection between malaria and sickle-cell anemia was not realized until the 1940's. This disease is found primarily in black populations in West Africa and their descendants (such as Afro-Americans). Linus Pauling first showed that sickle-cell anemia was a molecular disease resulting from the presence in the blood cells of an altered form of hemoglobin (hemoglobin S). Although sickle-cell anemia is a serious disease, it is less critical for human populations living at low altitudes, such as West Africa, than in other parts of the world. Thus, a person with sickle-cell trait can survive with little difficulty. It appears that sickle-cell trait confers on the person who has it a resistance to malaria, and such resistance would be of survival value in a region of the world where malaria is endemic, such as West Africa.

One of the most important advances in molecular genetics was the discovery by Vernon Ingram that hemoglobin S differed from normal hemoglobin A in a single amino acid in one of the hemoglobin polypeptides. Because sickle-cell anemia was known to be inherited as a single gene, Ingram's discovery showed that there was a one-to-one correspondence between a gene and the protein that it controls.

As discussed in this chapter, red blood cells that contain hemoglobin S are not as favorable for the growth of the malaria parasite as those containing hemoglobin A. In another region where malaria is endemic, the eastern Mediterranean, resistance to the malaria parasite is associated with a different change in red blood cells, a deficiency of the enzyme glucose-6-phosphate dehydrogenase. It thus appears that the malaria parasite has actually been an important agent in biochemical evolution of human populations.

An understanding of how the malaria parasite grows in the blood may aid in developing control methods for this serious disease. Despite control of the mosquito and the development of chemotherapeutic agents, malaria is still one of the most serious diseases of humans. In the long run, the most effective way of eliminating the disease would be by vaccination. In Chapter 9, "The Molecular Approaches to Malaria Vaccines," the possibility of using biotechnology to develop a malaria vaccine is described.

Molecular Approaches to Malaria Vaccines

Study of genes encoding the molecules of the malaria parasite's outer coat reveals a class of proteins forming repeated antigenic sites. They may serve as decoys deflecting the immune response.

· · ·

G. Nigel Godson
May, 1985

For a brief period in the early 1960's it appeared that malaria, an ancient scourge, might soon be brought under control. Extensive spraying with DDT was reducing the *Anopheles* mosquito population and novel drugs such as chloroquine were available for treating infected patients (see Postscript to Chapter 8, "The Biochemistry of Resistance to Malaria").

Twenty years later malaria is resurgent. Its causative agent, the protozoan parasite *Plasmodium*, is developing resistance to the drugs, and the parasite's vector, the female *Anopheles* mosquito, is becoming resistant to DDT and other insecticides. Today the disease afflicts some 200 to 400 million people in a broad tropical band around the world. In Africa it kills some 10 percent of its victims directly and debilitates the rest; it is a major cause of early-childhood mortality rates ranging as high as 50 percent. Clearly there is urgent need for the new attack on malaria that is currently under way. The major effort is to exploit the tools of molecular biology to develop antimalaria vaccines and other ways to combat the parasite.

An effective vaccine must stimulate the immune system to make antibodies that can attack and neutralize the parasite. To develop such a vaccine will not be easy. In regions of Africa where the disease is endemic a large proportion of the population is either chronically infected with one or another species of the parasite or is continually reinfected by the ever-present mosquito. These people develop antibodies aplenty to the parasite, but few of them develop protective immunity. The reason is that *Plasmodium*, even during the brief periods when it is not hidden from the immune system of its human host (in liver cells or red blood cells), is adept at evading the immune response. Studies of the molecular biology of *Plasmodium* have begun to reveal how it does so and to suggest new approaches whereby the parasite's escape mechanisms may be circumvented. One can hope that in the not too distant future genetically engineered vaccines or other molecular weapons may be developed and that eventually malaria will be eradicated.

Two species of *Plasmodium* are important agents of human malaria: *P. falciparum* (the most prevalent and most lethal) and *P. vivax*. In the course of its life cycle in its mosquito and human hosts the unicellular parasite undergoes an astounding series of developmental and morphological changes (see Figure 9.1). The stage that infects humans, the

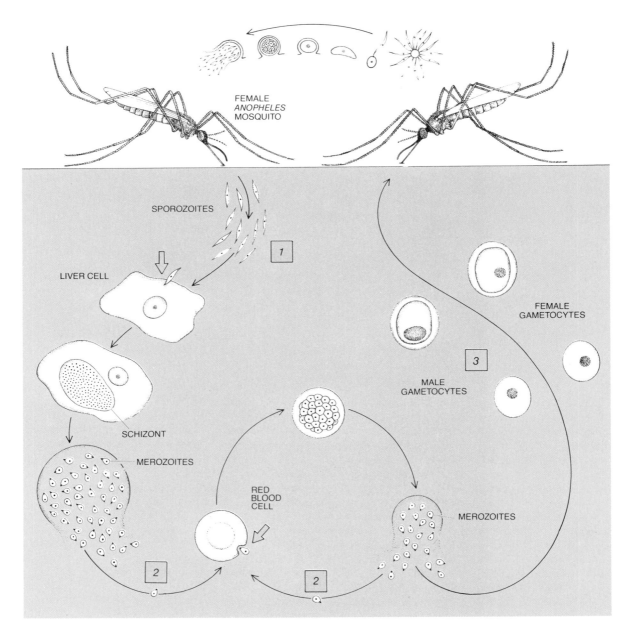

Figure 9.1 MALARIA PARASITE goes through a number of stages in a female *Anopheles* mosquito and in a mammalian host. A sporozoite injected by the mosquito invades a liver cell where it is transformed into a schizont, which fissions, and the liver cell releases many thousands of merozoites. Each merozoite invades a red blood cell and multiplies; the cell bursts, releasing merozoites that invade more blood cells. Some merozoites become male and female gametocytes (germ-cell precursors), which are taken up with a blood meal by a mosquito. After a series of further transformations mature sporozoites appear in the mosquito's salivary gland, where they are available to repeat the infective cycle. A vaccine might be designed to elicit antibodies that attack sporozoites, merozoites, or gametocytes when they are free in the bloodstream (1, 2, 3). Agents might be designed to block the invasion of liver or blood cells (*colored arrows*) or to kill parasites within a cell.

lance-shaped sporozoite, resides in the mosquito's salivary gland and is delivered into the victim's bloodstream when the insect takes a blood meal. Within an hour each sporozoite finds its way to a liver cell. There it undergoes a complex series of transformations. Eventually a giant multinucleate stage, the schizont, fissions into small, roughly spherical merozoites. The result is an enormous amplification of parasites: a liver cell infected by one sporozoite releases into the bloodstream from 5,000 to 10,000 merozoites.

Each merozoite invades a red blood cell, where it multiplies asexually until the cell bursts and releases from 10 to 20 new merozoites that go on to invade more red cells. It is the periodic lysis of the blood cells, with concomitant release of merozoites and toxic waste products, that causes the regular fevers and chills of malaria.

Some merozoites develop into male and female gametocytes (germ-cell precursors), thus initiating the parasite's sexual cycle. The gametocytes are sucked up with red cells by a mosquito, mature in the mosquito gut and fuse to form a zygote. The zygote undergoes yet another series of divisions, transformations and migrations; eventually a mature sporozoite appears in the salivary gland, ready to initiate a new infective cycle.

Each developmental stage of *Plasmodium* has its characteristic shape and distinctive set of functions; it inhabits a particular microenvironment and interacts with a specific target tissue. To the molecular biologist this means that although all the stages have the same genome, or complement of genes, in each stage a different part of the genome is being expressed: different genes are turned on and off in a programmed sequence.

A gene is composed of DNA, a double helix whose two complementary strands are made up of subunits called nucleotides. Each nucleotide is characterized by one of four bases: adenine (*A*), guanine (*G*), thymine (*T*) and cytosine (*C*). Genetic information is encoded in the sequence of the bases. A gene is expressed when one strand of its DNA is transcribed into a complementary strand of messenger RNA (mRNA), which is then translated into a sequence of amino acids, the subunits of proteins.

One way to understand a developing organism at the molecular level is to isolate the genes being expressed at a particular stage of development and study their structure and that of the proteins they encode. In the case of *Plasmodium* such studies have been focused on the parasite's surface. One reason

is that the proteins of the cell's outer coat are highly stage-specific: each is expressed in only a single developmental stage. Their genes must therefore be subject to stringent regulation, whose mechanisms are of considerable fundamental interest. The other reason is that these proteins are surface antigens and as such are likely to be implicated in triggering (or in evading) the host's immune response. Studying their genes is therefore important not only for understanding the mechanism of stage-specific gene expression but also for developing stage-specific malaria vaccines.

Some years ago my colleagues and I at the New York University Medical Center set out to isolate and study the gene encoding the major surface antigen of a sporozoite, the so-called circumsporozoite (*CS*) protein. The protein had been studied for many years by Ruth S. Nussenzweig of NYU and had been shown to be stage-specific: synthesized only in sporozoites. It is the major protein synthesized by sporozoites in the salivary gland and it covers the entire surface of the cell. We chose to work with *P. knowlesi*, the agent of monkey malaria, largely because the *Anopheles* species that carries it generates some 10 times as many sporozoites as a mosquito infected with one of the human parasites. Infected mosquitoes were supplied by Robert W. Gwadz and Louis H. Miller of the National Institute of Allergy and Infectious Diseases (NIAID), who provide many investigators worldwide with malaria-parasite material.

To isolate an active stage-specific gene one ordinarily begins with the total mRNA of the stage under study, and so we tested several laborious methods for separating sporozoite material from infected mosquitoes. Eventually we found that instead of having to purify sporozoites we could begin with the total mRNA of infected mosquitoes (or of their thoraxes). In the mixture of sporozoite and mosquito mRNA we could detect the specific mRNA encoding the *CS* protein, and so we could clone the parasite gene directly from the total mRNA.

The procedure we used is shown in Figure 9.2. The total mRNA was converted with the enzyme reverse transcriptase into a DNA copy (cDNA). The cDNA fragments were inserted into plasmids (small circles of bacterial DNA) in the middle of a gene coding for a plasmid protein. A recombinant plasmid incorporating the parasite cDNA should there-

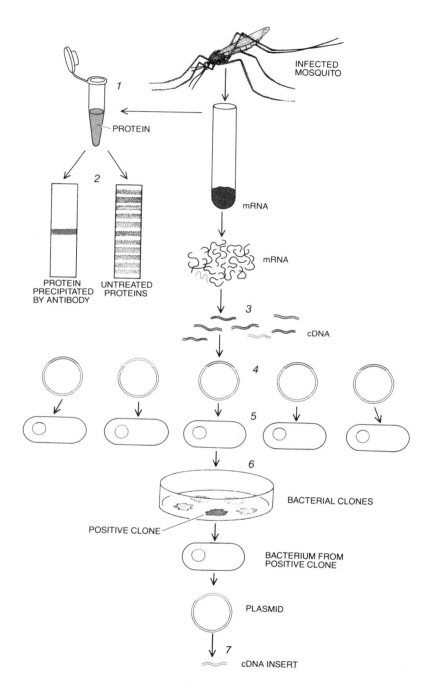

INFECTED MOSQUITO

PROTEIN

PROTEIN PRECIPITATED BY ANTIBODY

UNTREATED PROTEINS

mRNA

mRNA

cDNA

BACTERIAL CLONES

POSITIVE CLONE

BACTERIUM FROM POSITIVE CLONE

PLASMID

cDNA INSERT

Figure 9.2 SEARCH FOR GENE encoding *CS* protein of the malaria parasite. Some of the mRNA was translated into radioactively labeled protein (*1*). Half of the protein was subjected to precipitation with a monoclonal antibody to the *CS* protein (*2*). The presence of a band of protein that had been precipitated by the antibody (*color*) gave assurance that the *CS*-protein mRNA was present. The total mRNA was reverse-transcribed (*3*) into cDNA, which was inserted into plasmids (*4*). The recombinant plasmids were introduced into bacterial cells (*5*) and the bacteria were grown (*6*). Some resulting clones were found to have expressed the protein (*color*). Three plasmids in the positive clones were found to carry parasite-cDNA inserts coding for part of the sporozoite protein (*7*).

fore express a fusion product, part plasmid protein and part parasite protein.

Recombinant plasmids were introduced into the bacterium *Escherichia coli*. The bacteria were grown and the resulting clones (colonies descended from a single cell) were screened with the monoclonal antibody to the *CS* protein by means of a two-site immunological assay developed by Fidel P. Zvala of NYU. Joan Ellis, a student in my laboratory, found three clones to which antibody bound, showing that these bacteria had synthesized an active fusion protein.

When the plasmids in the positive *E. coli* clones were analyzed, we found that the fragment of sporozoite cDNA inserted in one of them was extremely short: only 340 base pairs, or long enough to encode only about 110 amino acids (since each amino acid is specified by a codon of three nucleotides). This was a serendipitous finding with remarkable ramifications. It meant that this small fragment of sporozoite cDNA must include the region of the gene coding for the immunoreactive part of the CS protein: the epitope, or antibody-combining site.

To locate the epitope-encoding region of the small cDNA insert more precisely we turned to transposon mutagenesis. This mapping technique depends on bacterial transposons: bits of DNA, often encoding a gene for antibiotic resistance, that can jump from one plasmid to another almost at random. A transposon inactivates gene function beyond the point at which it is inserted, so that by mapping the insertion sites that result in deactivation one can delimit functional regions of genes. By this means James R. Lupski, another student in the laboratory, was able to show that the antigen-combining site is encoded within a segment some 110 base pairs long at the extreme left-hand end (what is called the 5' end) of the 340-base-pair insert.

Pamela Svec then determined the nucleotide sequence of the 340-base-pair insert. To our astonishment the entire insert turned out to consist of tandem repetitions of a single sequence 36 base pairs long; there were seven complete repeat units, with incomplete units at each end. When the other two clones to which the CS-protein antibody had bound were examined (the ones in which the sporozoite cDNA inserts were larger), we found those inserts also incorporated multiples of the 36-base-pair unit. Since the repeat unit was common to all three positive clones, it seemed clear that it must code for the CS protein's epitope. The epitope itself must be a chain of 12 amino acids repeated in tandem—an entirely new and remarkable structure for a surface antigen (see Figure 9.3).

We still did not know the amino acid sequence of the epitope. We knew the sequence of nucleotides but could not translate it into a sequence of amino acids because we did not know the reading frame: the way in which the string of nucleotides should be divided into codons specifying amino acids. Because a codon is a triplet of nucleotides, there are three

potential reading frames in each strand of DNA, and so there are six possible reading frames in the double helix.

We established which was the coding strand and deduced the reading frame by finding the junction between the *Plasmodium* DNA and the known nucleotide sequence of the plasmid-protein gene. Knowing the reading frame, we could translate the nucleotide sequence to derive the 12-amino-acid sequence of the epitope. The logical next step was to assemble a synthetic peptide (a short protein chain) corresponding to the derived sequence and see if it could mimic the immune properties of the natural sporozoite surface protein.

David H. Schlesinger of NYU assembled amino acids to make both the 12-amino-acid epitope and a double-unit peptide 24 amino acids long. The immunological assay showed that the double-unit synthetic peptide did bind to the monoclonal antibody against the CS protein. In a competitive assay the single-unit synthetic peptide not only bound to the antibody but also in doing so blocked the antibody's normal binding to the sporozoite surface (see Figure 9.4). These results established conclusively that the 12-amino-acid peptide did either constitute the epitope of the *P. knowlesi* surface antigen or include it. The latter proved to be the case: in further experiments done with Victor Nussenzweig and Schlesinger we showed that synthetic peptides consisting of only eight of the 12 contiguous amino acids carry all the information needed for a complete antigen-antibody interaction.

At this point several advances had been made. The sequence of the epitope had been determined; the reading frame of the entire CS-protein gene had been established, and synthetic peptides had been constructed that mimicked the protein's immunoreactive region. When the peptides were injected into mice and rabbits, they were highly immunogenic, that is, they stimulated the formation of antibodies. Whether the antibodies would establish protective immunity (in which case the peptides could be the basis of an antimalaria vaccine) remained to be determined by testing in animals and by further studies of the molecular biology of the surface antigen.

The next objectives were therefore to establish the structure of the complete CS-protein gene (not a cDNA construct but the actual gene found in the parasite chromosome) and to deduce the complete amino acid sequence of the protein and then its structure. Luiz S. Ozaki fragmented the parasite's genomic DNA, separated the fragments according

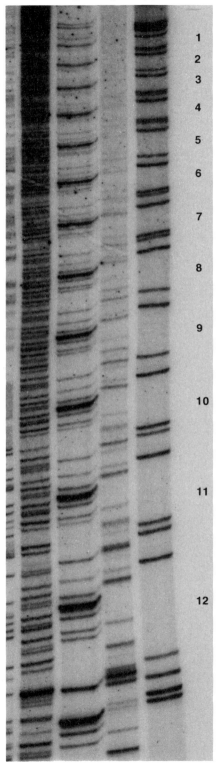

to size by electrophoresis and transferred them to a nitrocellulose filter (see Figure 9.5). He probed the filter with one of our plasmid cDNA's. The cDNA probe hybridized with (bound to) a complementary stretch of DNA contained within one segment, 11,000 nucleotides long, of the parasite genome. The gene for the CS protein was thereby shown to be within that segment.

After isolating the 11-kilobase fragment (by cloning) and establishing its overall structure (by restriction-enzyme mapping), we determined the full nucleotide sequence of the region containing the surface-antigen gene. The sequence of the entire CS-protein gene is illustrated in Figure 9.6. The mapping and sequence data led us to two conclusions. One was that, in spite of the vast amplification of CS-protein expression known to take place during the sporozoite stage, the parasite genome contains only one gene for the protein. The other conclusion was that the coding region of the gene, unlike most genes in eukaryotes (organisms higher than bacteria), is not interrupted by introns: noncoding intervening sequences that are removed only when the mRNA is processed. The lack of introns suggests that *Plasmodium* may be a very primitive eukaryote.

With the reading frame established and the full nucleotide sequence of the CS-protein gene in hand we could deduce the amino acid structure of the complete protein. The central 45 percent or so of the protein turned out to consist of 12 repeats of the 12-amino-acid epitope unit. In some respects other parts of the protein were what might be anticipated in a surface protein. The extreme left end (the NH_2 terminus) has the strongly hydrophobic (water-repellent) signal sequence characteristic of proteins exported through the outer membrane of a cell. The other end (the COOH terminus) is a hydrophobic tail (which typically anchors a surface protein in the cell membrane); it is preceded by four amino acids

Figure 9.3 REPEATED PEPTIDES were noted when the nucleotide sequence of a cDNA insert encoding the CS protein was being determined. The four columns of the autoradiograph represent occurrences of the four subunits (T, G, C, A) of which DNA is composed. Even before the sequence was read off it was evident from the reiterated pattern that this part of the gene encodes 12 tandem repetitions of a short peptide. The peptide is an epitope, or antigenic determinant: a specific site on the protein that binds to an antibody. The region of the protein encoded here is therefore a multiple epitope.

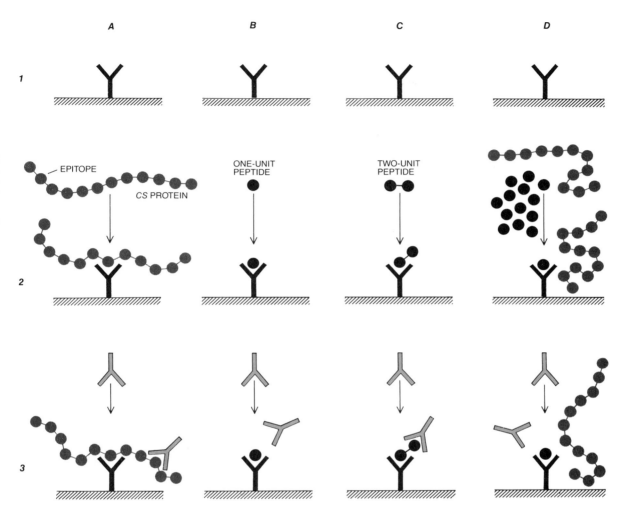

Figure 9.4 MONOCLONAL ANTIBODY to the *CS* protein serves to detect clones expressing the protein (*A*) and to test synthetic peptides and verify the deduced amino acid sequence of the epitope (*B–D*). Unlabeled antibody is adsorbed on a solid surface (*1*). A positive clone is detected (*A*) when an epitope on the *CS* protein it expresses binds to the antibody (*2*); binding of the protein is demonstrated by the binding of a labeled copy of the same antibody to a second epitope on the protein (*3*). When a single synthetic peptide binds to the adsorbed antibody (*B*), it offers no second site for attachment of the labeled antibody. The double peptide does provide a second site (*C*), and the labeled antibody can bind to it. In a competitive assay (*D*) the single peptide at high concentration saturates the combining sites of adsorbed antibodies and blocks the binding of the true *CS* protein.

(cysteines) between which disulfide bonds can form to link segments of the protein into a globular structure or to link adjacent molecules of the protein.

The protein's molecular weight as calculated from the amino acid sequence is, however, substantially less than the molecular weight measured by the protein's rate of migration in a gel. This finding and others suggested that the CS protein must have pe-

culiar physical properties. Some of these properties could be deduced from the amino acid sequence of the repeat unit. The peptide has three glycines, three alanines, three glutamines and an aspartic acid, a proline and an asparagine. They are arrayed in two dimensions in such a way that small polar (hydrophilic) amino acids alternate with large hydrophobic ones. Such alternation is also characteris-

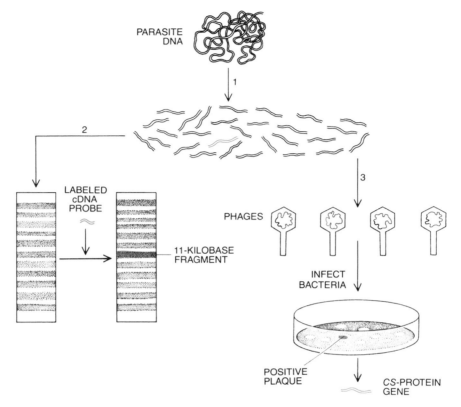

PARASITE DNA

LABELED cDNA PROBE

11-KILOBASE FRAGMENT

PHAGES

INFECT BACTERIA

POSITIVE PLAQUE

CS-PROTEIN GENE

Figure 9.5 ISOLATION OF THE entire *CS*-protein gene. The sporozoite genome (total DNA) was digested with an enzyme (*1*). The fragments were separated by size on a gel (*2*) and a labeled *CS*-protein cDNA insert was used as a probe to show that the gene was within a particular 11-kilobase fragment (*color*). That fragment was isolated by cloning (*3*). The DNA fragments were introduced into a bacterial virus, phage lambda. The phages infected bacteria cultured in a petri dish. Each phage multiplied, leaving a discrete plaque in the lawn of bacteria. With the labeled cDNA insert again serving as a probe, plaques containing the 11-kilobase fragment were identified. The *CS*-protein gene was isolated from a positive plaque.

tic in a six-amino-acid repeating subunit of fibroin, the major protein of silk. The fibroin chain doubles back and forth on itself, with successive antiparallel segments linked by hydrogen bonds. This configuration, a beta pleated sheet, gives silk its fibrous, flexible nature.

By building molecular models we showed that the CS protein's repeating peptides could form a similar pleated sheet. The peptide chain would bend at each proline (where protein chains often turn sharply), so that succeeding units of the repeat zigzag in opposite directions (see Figure 9.7). Hydrogen bonds form naturally; the sizes of the amino acids' side chains alternate in such a way that abutting side chains do not interfere with each other.

Such a beta sheet should be very stable. In collaboration with Schlesinger and Walter A. Gibbons of the University of London, we have recently confirmed some of the predictions of this proposed structure experimentally. When peptides corresponding to two, three and four tandem repeats (24, 36 and 48 amino acids) are synthesized, they do show considerable beta structure, strongly suggesting that this is the case in the natural protein.

If the repeats of a single *CS*-protein molecule can zigzag to form a sheet, adjacent molecules should be able to interact in a similar way (as they do in fibroin). This would make for a surface structure in which molecules fold on themselves and interact with one another to form a network: an ideal protective surface for the parasite (see Figure 9.8). It is

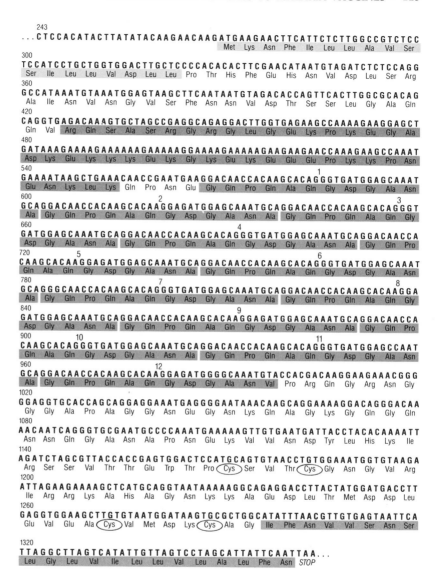

Figure 9.6 NUCLEOTIDE SEQUENCE of the entire *CS*-protein gene was determined. The protein has a hydrophobic signal region (*yellow*), which promotes its passage through the sporozoite's cell membrane, and a region of basic amino acids (*green*). Then comes the antibody-binding region (*red*): 12 tandem repeats of a 12-amino-acid epitope. The sequences of the repeated epitopes are almost identical. Most of the few nucleotide differences, such as those in the triplets encoding the central glutamine (*Gln*) and glycine (*Gly*), do not result in amino acid changes; only the final valine (*Val*) is a substitution. Two pairs of cysteines, which can form disulfide bonds, precede the hydrophobic anchor region (*blue*).

more than a physical barrier. The *CS* protein appears to promote the sporozoite's evasion of the host's defenses primarily by "focusing" the immune response, concentrating it on a single target to the detriment of its ability to find other targets. Several lines of evidence point to such a strategy.

When an experimental animal is injected with sporozoites, most of the antibodies it raises are directed against the *CS* protein, and specifically against the repeating epitope; there is little indication that the immune system recognizes any other part of the surface protein. This suggests that the protein chain is folded so that only the 45 percent of the chain carrying the repeating epitope is exposed on the surface. Each molecule of the protein therefore presents to the immune system only one vulnerable site — but that site is repeated 12 times. The immune system sees multiple identical targets on

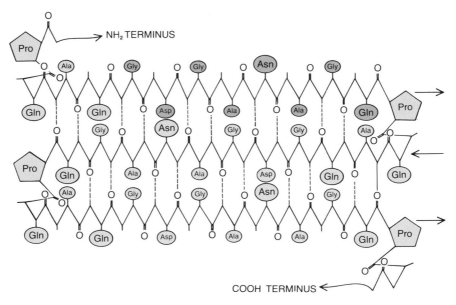

Figure 9.7 CONFIGURATION of the repeated-epitope region (the immune decoy) can be predicted from its amino acid sequence. It is likely to be an antiparallel beta pleated sheet, in which a polypeptide chain folds back and forth on itself and adjacent segments of the chain are linked into a sheetlike structure by hydrogen bonds (*broken lines*). The chain would fold by bending sharply at each proline (*Pro*). Both the size and the charge of abutting amino acids suggest they would not interfere with one another. Experiments have shown that eight contiguous amino acids (*dark color*) suffice to interact with the antibody to the *CS* protein.

the same molecule; any other potential targets are relatively inaccessible.

The repeating epitope, then, is essentially a multiple decoy. It is also a renewable decoy. Many years ago Jerome P. Vanderberg of NYU noted that sporozoites exposed to antisporozoite antibodies appeared to slough off a discrete surface coat. The coat is visible in electron micrographs as a thick, fuzzy layer surrounding the cell; presumably it is the network of *CS* protein molecules. There is evidence that the sporozoite's coat is sloughed off continually and is continually restored by newly synthesized protein secreted to the surface. It is notable that the *CS* protein is manufactured in large amounts, accounting for from 10 to 30 percent of the total protein synthesized by the sporozoite in the mosquito salivary gland. The immune system, then, is presumably forced to mount a larger than normal attack both because there are multiple epitopes and because the surface coat is continually replaced. Moreover, the sloughed-off molecules, particularly if they are present as a network, must act as a further decoy that tricks the immune system into recogniz-

ing them as live parasites and thus mops up still more antibodies.

All of this may give sporozoites injected by a mosquito time to reach shelter in liver cells even if circulating antisporozoite antibodies are already present in the host because of previous infection. Such an escape mechanism would be particularly appropriate for a parasite stage such as the sporozoite, which is exposed to the immune system only during a short interval. On the other hand, a parasite exposed to antibodies for a long time, such as the trypanosome, may need to keep changing its surface antigens so that the immune system cannot catch up with it (see Chapter 10, "How the Trypanosome Changes Its Coat"). Such antigenic variation takes time, however. An immune-decoy protein, on the other hand, can protect a parasite from the moment it appears in the host.

Soon after we described the surface antigen of the *P. knowlesi* sporozoite a remarkably similar one was isolated from a different stage (the blood-stage merozoite) of the human malaria parasite *P.*

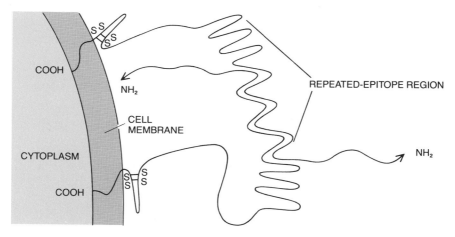

COOH

NH₂

CELL MEMBRANE

CYTOPLASM

COOH

REPEATED-EPITOPE REGION

NH₂

Figure 9.8 BETA SHEET providing an ideal protective surface for an invading parasite could be formed by both intramolecular and intermolecular interactions. The polypeptide chain of a *CS*-protein molecule could fold and be hydrogen-bonded to itself or to the folded chain of an adjacent molecule. The drawing suggests how molecules embedded in the parasite cell membrane might interact to form part of a network constituting the parasite's outer coat.

falciparum. Working with mRNA of the blood-form parasites and the serum of people repeatedly exposed to the parasite, David J. Kemp, Robin F. Anders and Graham F. Mitchell and their colleagues at the Walter and Eliza Hall Institute of Medical Research in Australia were able to clone and express a number of merozoite surface-antigen genes.

One of them was the gene for a merozoite *S* antigen, a surface protein that forms a fuzzy layer covering the merozoite as it emerges from a lysed red blood cell. As in our *CS*-protein gene, there is a multiple repeat. In the *S*-antigen gene the repetitive sequence is 33 base pairs long (so that it codes for a repeating peptide with 11 amino acids rather than 12) and the sequence is repeated in tandem more than 100 times (rather than 12 times). Like the *CS* protein, the *S* antigen seems to be an immune-decoy protein that is continually secreted and shed and presents a repeated epitope to the immune system.

Since the *P. knowlesi CS* protein and the *P. falciparum S* antigen were characterized, five more *Plasmodium* surface proteins have been isolated (see Figure 9.9). The work has been done by Kemp and his colleagues in Australia, by Miller's group at NIAID in collaboration with a group at the Walter Reed Army Institute of Research, by Jeffrey V. Ravetch of the Memorial-Sloan Kettering Cancer Center and Gunter Blobel of Rockefeller University and by Luis Pereira da Silva of the Pasteur Institute and Benno Müller-Hill of the University of Cologne. Every one of these proteins has a tandemly repeated peptide unit. Most of the repeating peptides include a proline, raising the possibility that zigzagging at a proline may give rise to a beta pleated sheet in all plasmodial surface antigens.

It seems clear that many of the major surface proteins of both sporozoites and merozoites are immune decoys and that the antibodies they induce are not protective ones; they do not incapacitate the parasite. That probably explains why natural infection rarely results in protective immunity. It also leads one to conclude that vaccines designed to stimulate antibodies against these major surface antigens are probably not the best candidates for inducing lasting immunity.

There may nonetheless be effective ways to attack the parasite. Judging by the multiplicity of antiplasmodial antibodies found in the blood of people with malaria, many more stage-specific surface proteins remain to be isolated and characterized. Most of them are probably directed against merozoites or against the surface of infected red blood cells (to which an infecting merozoite somehow exports some of its antigens), but some may be minor constituents of the sporozoite or gametocyte surface; unlike the major antigens, they are presumably not immune decoys. Many laboratories are engaged in

SPOROZOITES			
P. KNOWLESI	CS PROTEIN	Gly Gln Pro Gln Ala Gln Gly Asp Gly Ala Asn Ala (12)	
P. FALCIPARUM	CS PROTEIN	Asn Ala Asn Pro (41)	
BLOOD STAGES			
P. FALCIPARUM	S ANTIGEN	Pro Ala Lys Ala Ser Gln Gly Gly Leu Glu Asp (100-110)	
	RESA ANTIGEN	Glu Glu Asn Val Glu His Asp Ala	
	FIRA ANTIGEN	Val Thr Thr Gln Glu Pro	
	PF-11 ANTIGEN	Glu Glu Val Val Glu Glu Val Val Pro	
P. LOPHURAE	His-RICH PROTEIN	Ala Pro His$_8$ Asp Ala His$_8$	

Figure 9.9 SEVEN SURFACE PROTEINS of various *Plasmodium* species and stages have been isolated and characterized. All of them have repeated epitopes, whose sequences are given here. The number of repeats is also indicated for the three proteins in which it is known.

an effort to isolate the genes encoding these minor surface antigens by exploiting cloning procedures such as those described above. The problem will then be to learn whether any of them induce protective antibodies.

Clearly the parasite is most vulnerable when it is free in the bloodstream, seeking a target liver cell or red blood cell. There are three such stages at which a vaccine can be effective. An antisporozoite vaccine would be ideal: it would break the link between mosquito and man by stimulating the manufacture of antibodies able to attack the sporozoite at the initiation of infection, before it can reach the liver cells. An antimerozoite vaccine would stimulate an attack on the parasite in midinfection; in conjunction with an antisporozoite vaccine it would establish a second line of defense. An antigametocyte vaccine would break the link between man and mosquito.

There may also be ways to attack the parasite when it is not free in the bloodstream. The most likely opportunity may present itself during the invasion of a liver cell or a red blood cell. To recognize and enter these cells the parasite must detect and exploit some specific receptor on the target cell's surface. The sporozoite or merozoite may be equipped with a recognition molecule or, as Vanderberg has suggested, it may pick up from the host's serum a glycoprotein that serves this purpose. Once the molecular details of the invasion process are understood it may be possible to develop an analogue of the recognition molecule or an antibody to the cell's receptor molecule. Either one might bind to the receptor and thus block invasion. When the precise route of invasion is known, it may even be possible to develop an agent that will kill the parasite while it is inside a liver or blood cell.

The molecular study of *Plasmodium* is still in its infancy, but it has already yielded insights leading to new ways of thinking about the parasite and suggesting new ways to combat it. On the one hand, a molecular approach at the level of DNA seeks to identify mechanisms peculiar to the malaria parasite, one or more of which may prove to be an Achilles' heel. On the other hand, the power of molecular biology lies in the recognition that fundamental mechanisms of gene expression and cellular structure are common to all forms of life, and that what is learned in one biological system is applicable to all systems. Important advances in medicine apply new understanding of general mechanisms to solve specific medical problems, but at the same time they develop information that contributes to the expansion of fundamental knowledge.

POSTSCRIPT

As discussed in the Postscript to Chapter 8, "The Biochemistry of Resistance to Malaria," malaria is one of the most widespread diseases of humans, occuring especially in peoples in the tropical parts of the world. Although its mosquito vector has been controlled by DDT and the disease itself can be treated by quinine and its derivatives, there has never been a vaccine for malaria. Why is this so? This is in part because of the rather complex life cycle of malaria, involving both human and mosquito hosts, but mainly it is because the malaria parasite is an obligate parasite that can not be cultured readily in the large-scale equipment needed for the production of a vaccine. With the advent of the new biotechnology, the possibility of a malaria vaccine can be seriously considered.

In considering approaches to developing a malaria vaccine, it is important to understand how a vaccine works. The body forms antibodies against the various proteins of the parasite, but not all antibodies formed will confer immunity. An immunity-conferring antibody is one that will combine with an essential antigen on the surface of the parasite and alter this antigen in such a way that the parasite is no longer active. Since there are many antigens on the surface of the parasite, the problem is to find the right one. Once this antigen has been discovered, the gene for the antigen can be cloned, using recombinant DNA techniques. Once the gene is cloned into an appropriate cloning organism, such as the bacterium *Escherichia coli*, it is then possible to obtain the production of the antigen in the bacterium. It is relatively easy to grow *E. coli* in industrial-size equipment and commercial production is therefore possible.

In this chapter the techniques for cloning and expressing malaria antigens are laid out. Although the molecular study of the malaria parasite is still in its early stages and an effective vaccine has not yet been produced, it appears that given sufficient research effort, an effective vaccine will eventually become available. In Chapter 7, "Synthetic Vaccines," work on the production of completely synthetic vaccines is described. It would also be possible to produce a malaria vaccine by strictly chemical methods, but because of the large size of the antigen, synthetic production would be complicated and the cost prohibitive. By cloning the gene in a bacterium and letting the bacterium do the work, a much more economic approach is possible.

Probably the most significant result of the present work is the extensive new information it has led to on the immunology of malaria. Even though the malaria parasite is an obligate parasite and difficult to work with, quite sophisticated information can now be obtained using the techniques described in this chapter.

How the Trypanosome Changes Its Coat

The parasite, which deprives much of Africa of meat and milk, survives in the bloodstream by evading the immune system. Its trick is to switch on new genes encoding new surface antigens.

. . .

John E. Donelson and Mervyn J. Turner
February, 1985

The African trypanosome is a microscopic animal, a protozoan, that spends part of its life cycle as a parasite in the blood of human beings and other mammals. There it causes a fatal neurological disease, trypanosomiasis, whose final stage in humans is sleeping sickness. The disease is endemic in a vast region of Africa defined by the range of the tsetse fly, the intermediate host that carries the trypanosome from one mammalian host to another. About 50 million people are at direct risk of contracting the disease; some 20,000 new cases are reported every year and thousands of other cases no doubt go unreported. Even more important than the direct threat to human beings is the fact that domestic livestock are susceptible to trypanosomiasis. Between them the trypanosome and the tsetse fly make some four million square miles of Africa—an area larger than that of the U.S.—uninhabitable for most breeds of dairy and beef cattle (see Figure 10.1). Having little or no access to meat or dairy products, most of the human population is malnourished and susceptible to other diseases.

The key to the trypanosome's success is its ability to circumvent the mammalian immune system. A mammal ordinarily defends itself against viruses, bacteria or protozoa such as trypanosomes by manufacturing specific antibodies directed against the antigens, or "nonself" molecules, it recognizes on the foreign organism's surface; the antibodies bind to the antigens and neutralize or kill the invading organism. Some antibody-producing cells persist in the bloodstream and provide lasting immunity. Such immunity can also be elicited by a vaccine that mimics a natural infection (see Chapter 7, "Synthetic Vaccines").

Neither the immune response to infection nor vaccination can protect against trypanosomal infection. Even though these parasites are continually exposed in the bloodstream to the mammalian immune system (unlike the malaria parasite, discussed in Chapter 8, "The Biochemistry of Resistance to Malaria," and Chapter 9, "Molecular Approaches to Malaria Vaccines," which spends most of its life cycle sequestered within cells), they have evolved a way to evade the host's defenses: they keep changing the antigen that constitutes their surface coat. By the time the immune system has made new antibodies to bind to new antigens, some of the trypanosomes have shed their coat and replaced it with yet

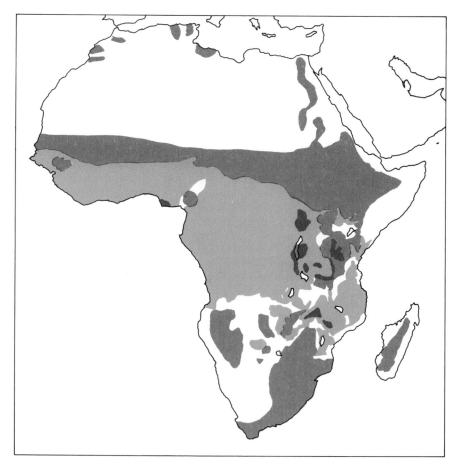

Figure 10.1 TSETSE FLY AND PARASITE together make some four million square miles of potential grazing land in Africa uninhabitable for most livestock. There is virtually no overlap between the range of the tsetse fly (*color*) and the cattle-raising regions of Africa (*gray*).

another antigenically distinct one. The host's overworked immune system is unable to cope with the infection, and so the parasites proliferate.

The molecular basis of this remarkable antigenic variation is under intensive study in a number of laboratories in Africa, Europe and the U.S. What has been learned suggests that there may be no way to help the immune system deal with trypanosomes once the parasites are established in the mammalian bloodstream, but that there may be other approaches to prevention or treatment.

The parasites that have evolved this very effective defense strategy are unicellular protozoans ranging from 15 to 30 thousandths of a millimeter in length. There are a number of species, which are classified on the basis of morphology and the hosts they infect. The two important species that infect human beings are *Trypanosoma rhodesiense* and *T. gambiense* (named for the colonial territories where they were first identified). Three species are important for their infection of livestock: *T. congolense*, *T. vivax* and *T. brucei*. Because it is easy to grow in laboratory animals and cannot survive in human blood, *T. brucei* is the preferred species for investigation.

Trypanosomes, like many other parasites, assume different forms at different stages of their complex life cycle. The trypanosomes ingested by a tsetse fly along with an infected mammal's blood lodge in the fly's midgut, where they begin to undergo a series of biochemical and structural changes (see Figure

10.2); in the process they lose their surface coat. After about three weeks they appear in the fly's salivary glands as the metacyclic form, which again carries a surface coat.

When the fly bites a mammal, metacyclic trypanosomes are introduced into the host's bloodstream, where they rapidly differentiate to a form that can proliferate. In humans the resulting disease can be either acute or chronic, depending on the infecting species. In both forms the disease first affects the blood vessels and lymph glands, causing intermittent fever, a rash and swelling. It is at this stage that the continuing battle with the host's immune system begins. Later the parasites invade the central nervous system; inflammation of the outer membranes of the brain leads to lethargy, coma and ultimately death.

The first indication that something keeps changing in the course of a trypanosome infection came early in this century. Physicians had observed a marked periodicity in the temperature of patients with trypanosomiasis. In 1910 the English investigators Ronald Ross and David Thomson, examining blood specimens taken from a patient every few days, noted that the changes in temperature were paralleled by a sharp rise and fall in the number of parasites in the blood. In reporting this finding Ross and Thomson quoted a suggestion, made by an Italian physician named A. Massaglia the year before, that "trypanolytic crises are due to the formation of anti-bodies in the blood. A few parasites escape destruction because they become used or habituated to the action of these antibodies. These are the parasites which cause the relapses." It was to be more than 50 years before this perceptive early insight could be confirmed and explained.

The explanation began to emerge in 1965, when Keith Vickerman of the University of Glasgow first described the thick surface coat covering the parasite's cell membrane. Soon it was discovered that individual trypanosome clones (populations descended from a single ancestral cell) have different surface coats (see Figure 10.3). In 1968 Richard

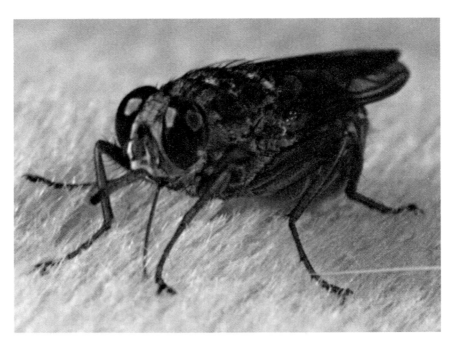

Figure 10.2 TSETSE FLY, the vector of the trypanosome that causes African sleeping sickness. The fly's proboscis and distended abdomen are red with blood ingested from an experimental animal in this photograph made by Edgar D. Rowton of the Walter Reed Army Institute. The fly is not only the vector but also the intermediate host, and the parasite goes through several developmental stages before it is injected into a mammalian host.

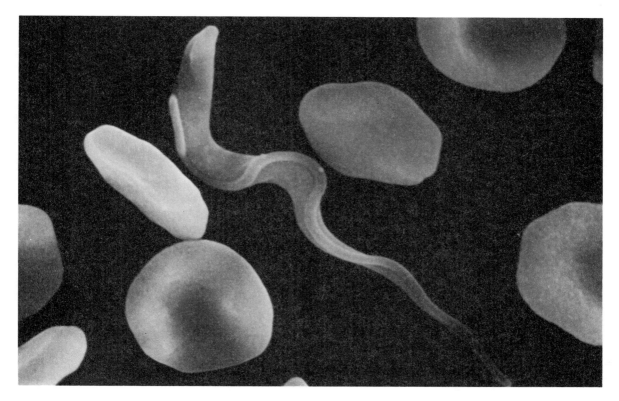

Figure 10.3 TRYPANOSOME and red blood cells are enlarged 5,500 diameters in this scanning electron micrograph made by Steven T. Brentano of the University of Iowa. The parasite, which is introduced into a mammal's bloodstream by the bite of the tsetse fly, is a unicellular animal (a protozoan) with a single flagellum extending along one side. The parasite's surface is covered with variable surface glycoproteins (VSG's). They are antigenic: the mammal's immune system makes antibodies that bind to them, killing the parasite. A trypanosome can change its surface coat, however, giving rise to a new parasite population that evades the host's antibody defense.

W. F. Le Page of the Medical Research Council's Molteno Institute in Cambridge, England, analyzed the antigenic surface proteins isolated from a number of clones. He found that each clone displayed a biochemically different protein; the differences were so marked that they suggested each antigen must represent the expression of a different gene. (A gene is expressed by a cell when the DNA of the gene is transcribed to make a strand of messenger RNA, which is subsequently translated to make a protein.)

During the mid-1970's George A. M. Cross and his colleagues at the Molteno Institute generated four different clones from a trypanosome population infecting a laboratory animal. They showed that the surface coat consists of a matrix of identical glycoprotein molecules (proteins to which carbohydrate groups are attached) and that the glycoproteins are the same in all individuals in a single clone. Having determined the sequence of the amino acids (the subunits of protein chains) at the beginning of the glycoproteins of their four clones, they noted that the sequence was different in each case; the observation supported Le Page's proposal that different surface antigens must be encoded by different genes. These antigens are now called variable surface glycoproteins, or VSG's (see Figure 10.4).

Early in the course of an infection the immune system generates antibodies shaped to bind to the particular VSG's it "sees" on the surface coat of invading parasites. The antibodies kill perhaps 99 percent of the original parasite population. A few

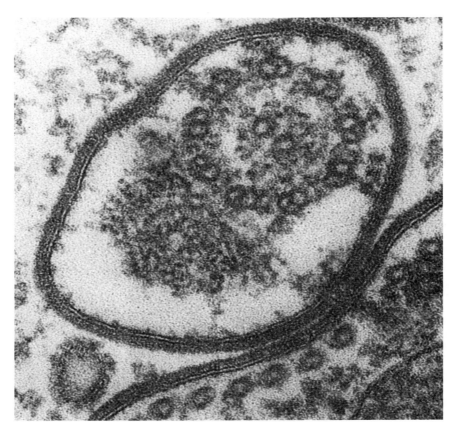

Figure 10.4 TRYPANOSOME'S SURFACE COAT of VSG's is visible as a diffuse, dark layer in an electron micrograph made by Laurence Tetley and Keith Vickerman of the University of Glasgow. A cross section of the parasite's body and flagellum has been enlarged about 190,000 diameters. The double membrane just inside the surface coat is the cell membrane.

individual trypanosomes escape, however, because they have turned on a different VSG gene and are covered by a new coat of VSG's to which the available antibodies cannot bind (see Figure 10.5). These variant individuals give rise to a new population expressing the new set of VSG's; the new population grows while the immune system raises another set of antibodies, which eventually succeed in again killing some 99 percent of the parasites. By that time, however, a few of the parasites have changed their coat again, and therefore a new population proliferates. So it goes until the host dies. The available evidence suggests that the switch from one VSG to another takes place spontaneously. The host's immune system does not induce the switch but rather selects (by its inability to deal quickly with a particular new antigen) a variant that initiates a new population (see Figure 10.6).

The total potential VSG repertory of a trypanosome is not known. In controlled experiments trypanosomes derived from a single parent cell have generated more than 100 distinct VSG's, giving no indication that their complement of VSG genes has been exhausted. It has recently been estimated that a single organism has at least a few hundred and perhaps as many as 1,000 or so VSG genes. (This means that from 5 to 10 percent of the parasite's total genetic capacity is devoted to antigenic variation.) In the wild the combined gene pool of all trypanosomes probably supplies genetic information to generate a virtually infinite number of antigenically distinct VSG's.

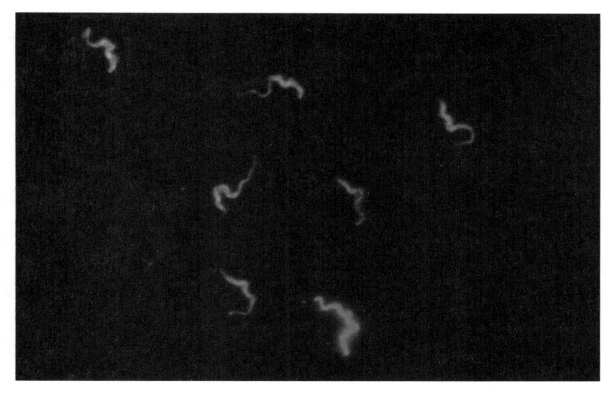

Figure 10.5 ANTIGENIC VARIATION is made visible in this double-exposure fluorescence micrograph made by Klaus M. Esser of the Walter Reed Army Institute of Research. Most of the trypanosomes are green because the antibody that recognizes and binds to their surface VSG has been labeled with a dye that gives off a green glow under ultraviolet radiation. One parasite is red. It has changed its surface coat and carries a different VSG, which is recognized by a different antibody: one that is linked to a red fluorescent dye.

What is the structure of the VSG and how is it attached to the cell membrane? How does the parasite manage to express one VSG gene at a time (and only one) out of a repertoire of hundreds of such genes? In order to learn something about the VSG's and about how they are displayed sequentially by the trypanosome, a number of research groups have been exploiting procedures based on recombinant-DNA technology.

The first step is to isolate the messenger RNA (mRNA) from a trypanosome clone. The procedure used is similar to that shown for malaria in Figure 9.2. The mRNA is copied to make what is called complementary DNA (cDNA), which is combined with a carrier DNA and introduced into bacteria. By manipulating the bacteria harboring the recombinant DNA, it is possible eventually to iso-

late a cDNA molecule that is in effect a copy of the VSG gene the trypanosome clone is expressing. By determining the sequence of nucleotides (the components of DNA) in the cDNA and translating it according to the genetic code, it is possible to predict the amino acid sequence of the VSG the gene encodes.

Partial or complete nucleotide sequences have been determined for some 15 cDNA's, and analysis of the deduced amino acid sequences reveals that each newly synthesized VSG is made up of about 500 amino acids. The first 20 or 30 of them at the N terminal of the protein constitute a signal peptide (a short protein chain) whose function is to help move the nascent VSG across the trypanosome's cell membrane; comparison of the cDNA-predicted amino acid sequence with the actual sequence of a few VSG's has shown that in the process the signal

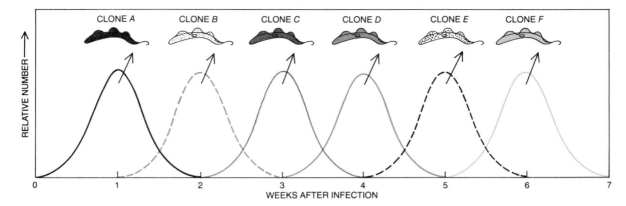

Figure 10.6 SUCCESSIVE WAVES of parasite proliferation in the blood resulting from antigenic variation. A population of parasites, some of which carry a particular antigen, VSG A, proliferates in the bloodstream for a few days. The immune system raises antibodies against the population's antigens, killing most of the parasites. A few individual parasites survive by expressing new VSG genes that direct the synthesis of new antigens, such as VSG B; these parasites give rise to a new population that grows until the immune system manages to raise new antibodies against the new antigens. The cycle is repeated many times in the course of a chronic infection. From each successive population it is possible to isolate individual trypanosomes and from them to grow clones expressing particular VSG's.

peptide is cleaved off (see Figure 10.7). The sequence of the next 360 amino acids is quite different in most VSG's, and this variable region is presumably responsible for the parasite's antigenic diversity. The last 120 amino acids (at what is called the C-terminal end of the protein) are quite similar in various VSG's; on the basis of the degree of similarity in these homology regions, VSG's can be classified into two homology groups.

Ordinarily it is peptide sequences in the C-terminal region of a surface protein that anchor the protein in the cell membrane, but the VSG is different. The last 20-odd amino acids of the region are clipped off in the mature VSG and are replaced by a structure containing an unusual oligosaccharide (a complex sugar molecule) that has a role in the anchoring. It seems to be very similar in all VSG's, regardless of their variable-region sequence, because antibodies raised against one oligosaccharide bind to all VSG molecules. Why does this cross-reacting determinant, as it is called, not induce natural immunity and why can it not serve as the basis of a vaccine? The reason is essentially that VSG's are packed into the surface coat in such a way that the immune system is confronted by the variable domain of the protein; the homology domain, including the cross-reacting determinant, is not exposed.

The cross-reacting determinant appears to be part of a larger oligosaccharide molecule, which is linked in turn to a phosphoglyceride carrying two fatty acid chains. It is the fatty acids that penetrate the cell membrane and hold the VSG in place (see Figure 10.8). Why would the trypanosome substitute this complicated structure for the usual C-terminal cell-membrane anchor? The reason may be that the ability to release its surface coat rapidly is of central importance to the parasite. The trypanosome has an enzyme that can cleave the link to the fatty acids, thereby releasing the VSG from the membrane. Having the same specialized anchoring molecule, subject to cleavage by the same enzyme, on all VSG's regardless of their exact sequence provides a rapid and universal mechanism for stripping off one coat and substituting another.

Although comparison of cDNA sequences has revealed extensive differences among VSG's, it has become clear that a very few amino acid changes can suffice to generate antigenically distinct VSG's. Presumably these changes take place at particular antigenic sites within the 360-amino-acid variable region. To find these sites it will be necessary to know the three-dimensional structure of the variable region in detail. Some progress toward that goal has come recently from X-ray-crystallographic

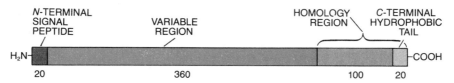

Figure 10.7 PROTEIN CHAIN of a typical VSG is composed of about 500 amino acids. The first 20 or so of these, at what is called the N terminal of the protein, constitute a signal peptide, which is cleaved from the protein before the VSG is implanted in the cell membrane. The next 360 amino acids (*color*) constitute the variable region, which is different in each antigenically distinct VSG. The final 120 amino acids at the C terminal are quite similar in each of two "homology groups" of VSG's. The last 20 amino acids of this region are cleaved from the chain and replaced by a large molecule that anchors the VSG in the cell membrane.

studies done by Don C. Wiley, Douglas M. Freymann and Peter Metcalf of Harvard University, in collaboration with one of us (Turner) at the Molteno Institute.

Five VSG's have been crystallized to date, but most progress has been made in determining the structure of the variable domain prepared from one of them. The resolution so far attained is enough to reveal the parts of a protein chain that are folded into the cylinder-like conformation known as an alpha helix. About half of the variable-region turns out to be in that form (see Figure 10.9).

The variable region crystallizes as a dimer (a double molecule made up of two monomers), and indeed VSG's seem to aggregate as dimers in the surface coat of a living trypanosome as well. The dimer (or at least the resolved half of it) is shown by crystallography to be a bundle of alpha helixes. The core of the bundle is made up of two hairpinshaped structures, one from each of the component monomers. At one end of the dimer the core interacts with two more helixes to form a six-helix bundle; at the other end the monomers diverge somewhat to form a distinctive head. This highly symmetrical structure must form the framework for the remaining half of the variable-domain sequence, unrevealed so far because it is not an alpha helix. We still do not know how the framework structure is oriented in the membrane (that is, which end is "out"), and so we cannot begin to guess where on the structure the major antigenic sites will be found.

Just what goes on when the trypanosome turns on one VSG gene after another, always synthesizing only one antigenically distinct surface glycoprotein at a time? Experiments designed to answer that question depend again on cDNA's of the kind described above. Now each such cDNA, which is in effect an artificial VSG gene, serves as a probe with which to locate copies of the same gene wherever they may be in the trypanosome genome (the total complement of genetic material).

The total genomic DNA is digested with a restriction enzyme, which cleaves the DNA at a specific site within a particular sequence of nucleotides. The result is that the genomic DNA is broken down into a large number of small fragments, each one slightly different in size. Having been separated according to their size by a process called gel electrophoresis, the fragments are transferred to nitrocellulose paper, to which they bind tightly. A cDNA representing a VSG gene, labeled with a radioactive isotope, is applied to the paper. The cDNA hybridizes with (binds to) any similar sequences it finds among the restriction fragments on the paper. Unbound cDNA is washed away and autoradiography reveals the sites of hybridization. One can thus determine how many different copies there are in a given trypanosome clone of the gene represented by the cDNA probe and whether or not the gene is in a different part of the genome in different clones.

In this manner Piet Borst and his colleagues at the University of Amsterdam and Cross and his associates at the Wellcome Research Laboratories in England demonstrated that when some VSG genes are expressed, an extra copy of the gene is present in the genome. They called it an expression-linked copy. Étienne Pays and Maurice Steinert of the Free University of Brussels went on to show that the mRNA for the expressed VSG gene is actually transcribed from this copy rather than from the original (basic-copy) gene that gave rise to it. Further analysis revealed that an expression-linked copy is always at a particular kind of site: near a telomere (the end of a chromosome). In other words, a single

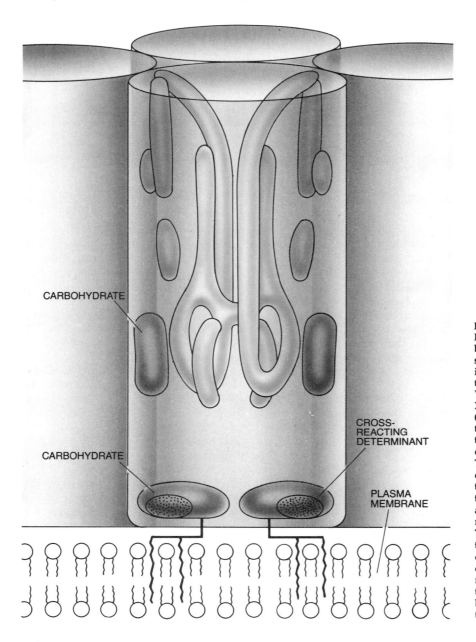

CARBOHYDRATE

CARBOHYDRATE

CROSS-REACTING DETERMINANT

PLASMA MEMBRANE

Figure 10.8 VSG'S OF SUR-FACE COAT may be assembled as indicated in this somewhat speculative drawing. The structure of part of the variable region of one VSG (*color*) is based on X-ray-crystallographic data (see Figure 10.9); the full extent of the VSG and the location of its neighbors are indicated by the gray cylinders. The variable region is a dimer, or double molecule, that appears to be a bundle of the protein structures called alpha helixes. Carbohydrate molecules flank the bundle. Two more carbohydrates at the base of the VSG may incorporate a small sugar molecule: the cross-reacting determinant. Fatty acids extending from these two carbohydrates appear to anchor the VSG in the membrane.

VSG gene out of the total repertory of such genes is expressed when it is duplicated and translocated to an expression site near a telomere; the switch from one VSG to another is often effected by the removal and degradation of one such copy and its replacement by the copy of another gene. The results of these studies are summarized in Figure 10.10.

This copy-and-translocate mechanism is not the only source of antigenic variation. John R. Young, Phelix A. O. Majiwa and Richard O. Williams of the International Laboratory for Research on Animal Diseases in Nairobi found another mechanism. They discovered that in some cases the number of different fragments to which a particular cDNA

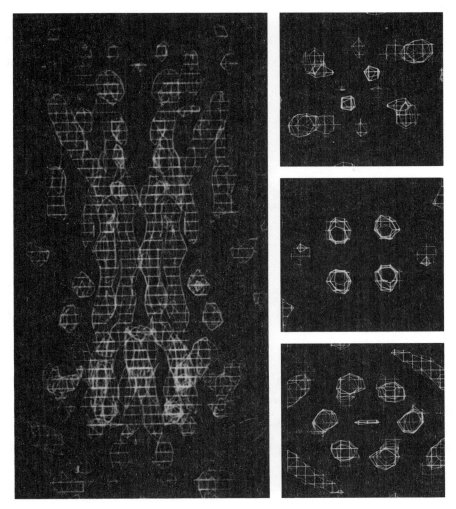

Figure 10.9 STRUCTURE of about half of a VSG's variable region was determined by X-ray crystallography. The region crystallizes as a dimer. An electron-density map (*left*), a view perpendicular to the axis of the dimer, reveals a bundle of rodlike alpha helixes. There are six helixes at one end (shown here as the bottom, although the actual orientation of the dimer is not known) and from four to six in the middle; the two monomers diverge at the top to form a two-headed structure. The three cross-sectional maps (*right*) are views along the dimer axis near the top, in the middle and near the bottom.

probe hybridizes does not change when the VSG gene represented by the probe is expressed: there is no expression-linked copy. The probe hybridizes instead to a fragment that is different in size in each trypanosome clone, whether or not the clone is expressing the gene.

What this means is that some VSG genes are expressed without being duplicated and translocated. These genes turn out to be already at a site near a telomere. Their proximity to a telomere explains why their fragments vary in size. In trypanosomes and in some other organisms it is often the case that a short DNA sequence is repeated hundreds of times near a telomere. The number of these "tandem repeats" between a VSG gene and a telomere varies from clone to clone. As a result the fragment carrying a given telomere-linked VSG gene can be a different size in different clones.

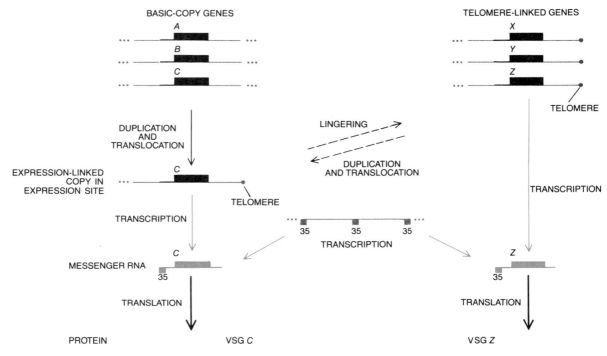

Figure 10.10 BASIC-COPY GENES in the interior of a try-panosome's chromosomes (*left*) are not ordinarily transcribed into messenger RNA (mRNA). For one of them (*C*) to be expressed it must be duplicated to provide an expression-linked copy. The DNA of the copy is translocated to an expression site near a telomere and is transcribed into mRNA, which is translated to make the VSG protein. Other VSG genes are already near a telomere (*right*). These telomere-linked genes can be expressed without forming an expression-linked copy, but occasionally they too are duplicated and translocated. An expression-linked copy is usually lost during an antigenic switch but sometimes "lingers" to become an unexpressed telomere-linked gene. Strangely, a 35-nucleotide sequence at one end of the mRNA is not encoded by the VSG gene but is specified instead by a separate region of repeated DNA.

About half of the VSG genes studied to date seem to be telomere-linked ones. Since there are hundreds of different VSG genes in the trypanosome genome, this suggests that there must be at least several hundred telomere-linked VSG genes in the genome, and so there must be hundreds of chromosomes in the parasite's nucleus! (The human chromosome complement is only 46.) Because the parasite has a normal amount of DNA for a unicellular animal, one would expect that some of the parasite's chromosomes must be very small, and indeed some of them are. A student of Borst's, Lex H. T. van der Ploeg, has applied a technique developed by David C. Schwartz and Charles R. Cantor of Columbia University to resolve trypanosomal nuclear DNA into four size classes: minichromosomes about 100,000 nucleotides long, other small chromosomes from two to seven times as long, mid-

dle-sized molecules (about two million nucleotides long) and others that are too long to be meaured by this method.

Van der Ploeg found VSG genes on chromosomes in every size class. In one case he found a basic-copy gene on a large chromosome and its corresponding expression-linked copy on a middle-sized one, indicating that translocation of a duplicated molecule can take place between chromosomes. In another case a telomere-linked gene was not duplicated but was expressed at its normal site near the end of a large chromosome. These observations supported earlier evidence, accumulated in several laboratories, that there must be more than one site in the genome at which VSG genes can be activated; they are not all translocated to the same unique expression site near a particular telomere. Although proximity to a telomere is necessary for expression, it therefore cannot be sufficient. Other factors must come into play that select and activate a single VSG gene in a given organism for transcription into mRNA at a given time.

Some of the events attending this activation may contribute to increasing the diversity of VSG's. Pays and Steinert and their colleagues have reported cases in which a functional expression-linked copy was generated not by the duplication of a basic-copy gene but by the "recombination" of segments of at least two different telomere-linked genes, each of which codes for a part of the resulting VSG. If this kind of recombination is a general phenomenon, it must enable the trypanosome to make even more VSG's than its hundreds of genomic VSG genes can specify. It also suggests a reason for the telomeric location of expression sites: highly repetitive stretches of DNA such as the short tandem repeats near telomeres are particularly likely to undergo recombination.

Occasionally an expression-linked copy is not destroyed during the switch to the expression of another gene but instead "lingers" for a while in its expression site. At the University of Iowa one of us (Donelson) has recently shown that the sequences at the boundaries of one particular expression-linked copy are virtually identical with sequences bounding a telomere-linked gene. This, together with similar findings from other groups, suggests that some telomere-linked VSG genes may be previously expressed expression-linked copies that have survived the switch to a new gene. Perhaps two chromosomes exchange regions adjacent to their telomeres, so that an expression-linked copy is removed from its original expression site and placed near a different telomere, where it is available for future expression. Perhaps, on the other hand, a single small segment of DNA in the genome serves as a mobile control element: an enhancer of transcription that can move from one telomere to another and cause different VSG genes to be expressed. In that case an expression-linked copy gene could remain in its expression site but be turned off by the control element's departure.

There is another peculiarity of trypanosomes and related organisms. The mRNA's for VSG's (and for many, if not all, other proteins) always begin with the same specific sequence of 35 nucleotides. This sequence is not found in the corresponding gene or anywhere in the DNA surrounding the gene. Instead it is coded for by a repetitive DNA sequence separated from the gene. Small RNA molecules

transcribed from this repeated DNA somehow provide copies of the 35-nucleotide sequence for the beginning of each mRNA. The 35-nucleotide sequence presumably has a role in the expression of trypanosome genes, but that role is not yet known.

Let us now summarize what is known about the mechanisms of antigenic variation in the trypanosome. There are hundreds of genes encoding VSG's in each organism's genome. They may be in the interior of chromosomes or near telomeres. Only one VSG is transcribed at a time, and that gene is always near a telomere. In order to be transcribed, an interior (basic-copy) gene needs to be duplicated and translocated (as an expression-linked copy) to one of many expression sites, all of which are near telomeres. A telomere-linked VSG gene, on the other hand, need not be duplicated in order to be expressed (although it may in fact sometimes be duplicated). Antigenic diversity may be further increased by recombination. The precise molecular mechanisms triggering the switch from one VSG gene to another are still not known. It would appear, however, that the mechanisms are so complex and varied that it is almost impossible to circumvent them, and so the development of a vaccine against trypanosomes in the bloodstream is unlikely.

It may, however, be possible to develop a vaccine against metacyclic trypanosomes. As we mentioned above, the metacyclic stage is the final developmental stage in the tsetse fly's salivary glands, and it is metacyclic parasites that are injected into the bloodstream when a fly bites a mammal. Steven L. Hajduk, J. David Barry and Vickerman at Glasgow and Klaus M. Esser of the Walter Reed Army Institute of Research in Washington found that the metacyclic parasites can display on their surface only a reduced subset of VSG's — perhaps as few as 15. Collaborating with Esser, one of us (Donelson) has studied the cDNA's of several metacyclic VSG's and shown that the proteins have about the same C-terminal homology region as bloodstream VSG's; apparently they attach to the cell membrane in the same way. Moreover, the genes for the metacyclic VSG's seem to be telomere-linked ones, like many of the bloodstream VSG genes. It is therefore not yet clear why metacyclic parasites cannot express the full range of VSG's. There may nonetheless be a way to take advantage of their limited repertory or of their switching mechanism in order to make an effective vaccine.

The drugs currently available for treating trypanosomiasis are extremely toxic and also cannot prevent reinfection, but new forms of chemotherapy may yet be found. The trypanosome cannot survive in a mammalian host without its surface coat; a drug that interferes with the phosphoglyceride anchoring the VSG in the cell membrane, or that activates the enzyme releasing the VSG, might therefore be an effective therapeutic agent. Mammalian messenger RNA's do not have the unusual 35-nucleotide sequence described above; a drug that interferes with its synthesis might therefore selectively disable the parasite. Drugs might also be found that act against two subcellular organelles that seem to be unique to trypanosomes. One is the glycosome, a membrane-bounded aggregation of enzymes; the other is the kinetoplast, an appendage of the parasite's single large mitochondrion. A drug interfering with a metabolic function of these organelles, or with some other unique metabolic pathway as yet undiscovered, might kill the trypanosome without harming its mammalian host.

There are some other possible approaches. The tsetse fly can be eradicated briefly in small areas by spraying with insecticides or by the distribution of sterile male flies, but such methods cannot be effective for a region that extends for some four million square miles and more than a score of countries. A few breeds of cattle herded by nomadic tribes do seem to have developed partial resistance to trypanosomiasis. They do not yield much meat or milk, but it may be possible to cross them with more productive breeds. It is also conceivable that wild animals such as the eland or the oryx, which seem not to be harmed by trypanosomes, might be domesticated and take the place of cattle.

The past few years have made it clear that African trypanosomes are superb experimental organisms. Continued investigation of their variable surface coat will provide basic information about such diverse subjects as the control of gene expression, the attachment and functioning of membrane proteins, the structure and replication of chromosomal telomeres and the molecular mechanisms that generate biological diversity.

Fundamental knowledge of this kind should in turn contribute to a truly pressing public health task: the control of trypanosomiasis. The next few years should show if new basic information about trypanosomes can be applied to control and perhaps eventually eradicate trypanosomiasis.

POSTSCRIPT

African sleeping sickness is one of the most serious and widespread diseases in Africa. It is caused by a flagellated protozoan of the genus *Trypanosoma*. Although primarily a disease of cattle, one species of the genus, *T. gambiense*, also infects humans. (There is also an American trypanosomiasis, Chagas disease, which is endemic in Central America and South America.) The connection between the tsetse fly, genus *Glossina*, and African sleeping sickness was first made by the British physician David Bruce early in the 20th century and methods to control the disease thus focused on the tsetse fly. However, control over the vast reaches of central Africa where the fly is native is extremely difficult, so that the disease remains rampant even today. Because the regions of Africa suitable for raising cattle are the same regions where the tsetse fly flourishes, the African cattle industry must continually struggle.

A vaccine for African sleeping sickness would clearly be a major economic development. Unfortunately, the trypanosome that causes African sleeping sickness has evolved a complex genetic mechanism for overcoming the immunity of the host, so that no sooner does an antibody against the parasite develop than the trypanosome has modified its surface structure so that it is resistant to the antibody.

Most of what is known about the antigenic structure and genetic variability of the trypanosome has been discovered using the recombinant DNA techniques. Because the trypanosome is an obligate parasite, its study in the laboratory has always been difficult, but by means of gene cloning it has been possible to pull out the genes responsible for the formation of the surface antigens and study their structure. Because there is a one-to-one correspondence between the base sequence in the DNA and the amino acid sequence in a protein, one can determine the amino acid sequence of a protein even if the protein has not been isolated, simply by determining the structure of the DNA. The trypanosome surface antigens have turned out to be complex proteins containing sugars (glycoproteins), and since they are highly variable they have been called variable surface glycoproteins or VSG's. The trypanosome has a whole array of VSG genes, and gene rearrangement can call into play any one of these genes.

It is important to emphasize that the antibody does not play a direct role in the expression of a VSG. The antibody acts simply as a selective agent, killing off trypanosomes that contain the reactive VSG and hence favoring the development of variants that produce different VSG's. Because of the vast array of VSG genes, it seems unlikely that a vaccine against VSG's will ever play a role in the prevention of African sleeping sickness.

However, antigens of the trypanosome exist other than the VSG's, and further research may lead to the development of an immunity-conferring vaccine against one of these. Hopefully, the fundamental knowledge being gained from modern studies on trypanosomiasis will eventually result in effective control of this widespread and extremely important disease.

THE PERILOUS ARM OF
INFECTIOUS DISEASE

. . .

Introduction to Section IV

In this section we present two quite diverse chapters that actually have a connection. Chapter 11, "Island Epidemics," deals with how epidemics spread, using data from some long-term studies of measles on the island of Iceland. Chapter 12, "The Birth of the U.S. Biological-Warfare Program," deals with the potential use of infectious agents for biological warfare. Although the motivation here is quite the obverse of the Iceland study, there is a connection because knowledge of how epidemics spread can be used to intentionally spread epidemics. Science is a two-edged sword, as these two chapters well demonstrate.

Island Epidemics

Epidemics are patterns in time and space that can best be perceived when they are studied in a small, isolated population. An example is provided by a study of a century of measles epidemics in Iceland.

· · ·

Andrew Cliff and Peter Haggett
May, 1984

Ever since Charles Darwin studied the finches of the Galápagos Islands in 1835 it has been recognized that oceanic islands can serve as large-scale laboratories for the investigation of biological processes. Not long after Darwin did his work it became clear that remote islands, which offer a simpler site for study than the crowded continental mainland, can also make a valuable contribution to the understanding of the spread of disease. In the late 1840's Peter Panum, a Danish physician, made a study of the 1846 measles epidemic on the Faeroe Islands that has become one of the classic works of epidemiology, the discipline concerned with the patterns of disease in human populations. Today most advances in the study of diseases caused by viruses are made in laboratories constructed by humans; for instance, the virus that causes measles was isolated in such a laboratory by John F. Enders and Thomas C. Peebles of the Harvard Medical School in 1954. Nevertheless, islands continue to play a significant role in the elucidation of how diseases spread under epidemic conditions.

An example of an island laboratory is the North Atlantic island of Iceland. The island republic has an area of about 40,000 square miles, roughly the same as that of Kentucky. It lies just south of the Arctic Circle, between 64 and 66 degrees north. The island is sparsely settled; its population has reached 200,000 only in recent years. Until air travel became common it was in an epidemiological sense isolated from many population centers in Europe. The most frequent contacts were with the Scandinavian countries, Denmark in particular. As a result of the severe winters residents of the island were isolated even from one another.

Since 1896 Iceland has had an unusually complete and trustworthy system of medical records that cover some 50 medical districts on a monthly basis. The combination of isolation, a small population and good medical records makes it possible to trace the pathways by which disease is transmitted in Iceland with more precision than such pathways can be traced in any other country.

The detail available in Iceland's public-health records could be employed to study many communicable diseases. Among the possible subjects measles is of particular interest for two reasons. The first reason is that measles is an excellent example of a disease that spreads rapidly in epidemic waves. It is highly infectious and readily recognized, and the epidemics tend to come at regular intervals. The second is that although in the U.S. measles has been all but eradicated by vaccination programs, it remains a serious threat to public health in the poorer countries of the world. In such countries the death rate in measles epidemics can be as high as 30 percent, particularly among children. Recent United Nations statistics show that in the world as a whole measles (and its complications) is one of the 10 most frequent causes of death.

Working with the unique public-health records of Iceland, we have shown that measles tends to spread in a hierarchical pattern according to the size of the community. As shown in Figure 11.1, measles moves from the capital city of Reykjavik to regional centers to villages and then to isolated farms. The records also show that when social and technological development changed the relations between the capital and the hinterland, the epidemiology of measles was profoundly altered. Such work could help in gaining an understanding of how the pathways along which measles spreads are determined. If the underlying factors are found, it might be pos-

sible to interrupt the pathways by selective programs of vaccination.

The virus that causes measles is a member of the family of paramyxoviruses, which includes the viruses that cause mumps and parainfluenza. When smallpox was eliminated after a long campaign (see Chapter 5, "The Eradication of Smallpox") and was dropped from the World Health Organization's list of infectious diseases in 1979, the attention of epidemiologists turned to other viruses. The measles virus became a prime candidate for elimination. One reason for thinking it could be eliminated is that if a community is small enough, the virus periodically disappears without any human intervention.

The periodic disappearance is due to the fact that in a small community the chain of measles infection is readily broken. Having measles confers a lifelong immunity to the virus, so that in such a community after a major epidemic the susceptible population is

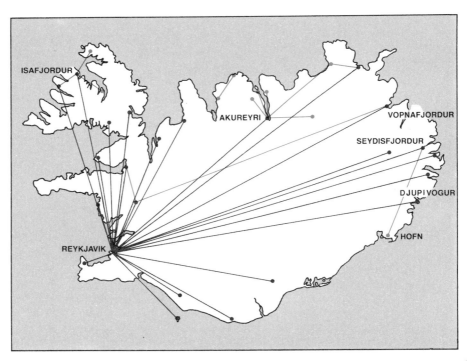

Figure 11.1 PATHWAYS OF TRANSMISSION for the measles virus in Iceland center on Reykjavik. The lines depict the routes followed by two or more cases in the 16 measles epidemics recorded from 1896 to 1975. Most of the frequently traveled pathways radiate from the capital (*black*). There are also small "circulation cells" around the provincial urban centers (*color*).

very small. Therefore even if the virus is present in the community, those who are infectious will not have contact with enough susceptible people for the chain of infection to remain unbroken. In a large community, on the other hand, the pool of those susceptible to the disease is large enough for some chains of infection to remain unbroken. As a result the virus is endemic, or continuously present.

How large must a human population be to maintain the measles virus on an endemic basis? Figure 11.2 contrasts measles epidemics in countries of different sizes. Maurice S. Bartlett of the University of Oxford concluded from his study of U.S. and British cities that between 4,000 and 5,000 reported cases of measles per year would suffice to sustain the disease continuously. Bartlett's work was done in 1957. The level of measles attacks and the rate of reporting of the disease to public-health authorities that then prevailed in the U.S. and the United Kingdom imply that 4,000 to 5,000 measles cases per year corresponds to a population of about 250,000. In a community with a population of less than 250,000 the virus apparently dies out, only to be reintroduced later by infected individuals coming from an area where infection is present. Large cities, where the disease is endemic, can serve as permanent reservoirs of infection. A person who introduces the virus into a small community where it was not present is called an index case. As we shall see, index cases are of much significance for tracing the pattern of measles epidemics.

It is clear that the pattern of epidemics in a small community depends on the frequency of contact between the small community and the larger centers of population where the virus is endemic. The frequency of contact in turn depends on the size of the small community, its distance from the big cities and the efficiency of the transportation networks that connect the small community and the large ones. If a community is small or remote, it will escape some of the epidemic waves that emanate at regular intervals from the cities.

Such demographic and geographic factors have enabled us to divide human communities into three groups. The division is done according to the form of the curve that traces the number of cases of measles in the community. The peaks in the curve correspond to epidemics. In large communities the curve has the form of a series of Type I waves (see Figure 11.3). Such waves are regular and continuous: between epidemics the number of measles cases never reaches zero. Medium-size communities

have Type II waves, which are regular but not continuous: between epidemics no measles cases are present. The smallest communities have Type III waves, which are discontinuous and irregular: because of their size and remoteness such communities miss some epidemics.

A decade after Bartlett's study Francis L. Black of the Yale University School of Medicine reexamined the relation between population size and epidemic waves but instead of working with cities he measured rates of infection in populations that are spatially even more isolated: the populations of 18 oceanic islands. Of the 18 islands only Hawaii, which then had a population of 650,000, showed the continuous Type I pattern. The Type II pattern was found on islands with a population as small as 10,000. Islands with fewer than 10,000 residents showed the Type III pattern.

After the work of Bartlett and Black a logical next step was to examine how measles spreads both between Type II islands and on a Type II island. For this purpose the 18 islands in Black's sample provided a convenient starting point. In the group of islands Iceland appeared to be the best laboratory for the work we planned to do (with J. K. Ord of Pennsylvania State University and the Icelandic health authorities).

Iceland is the largest island of the Type II group and has the second-largest population of the 18 islands. Its population is relatively small compared with the population of mainland regions, however, and the stern terrain and harsh climate of the interior have largely limited human settlement to the coastal lowlands. The coastline is deeply indented by fjords and the Icelandic communities tend to be remote from one another. Indeed, from an epidemiological point of view it is often appropriate to think of Iceland more as an archipelago than as a single island.

The Icelandic demographic records show that the population increased from fewer than 50,000 in the late 18th century to about 200,000 in 1970. About half of the population lives in Reykjavik and its suburbs, a fourth in the other 11 towns and the rest in the rural areas. The fourfold growth in population over the past two centuries has not been steady. The increase has been repeatedly interrupted by epidemics of infectious disease. The most potent of them was the smallpox epidemic that swept the island in the 1780's, but there were also, in addition

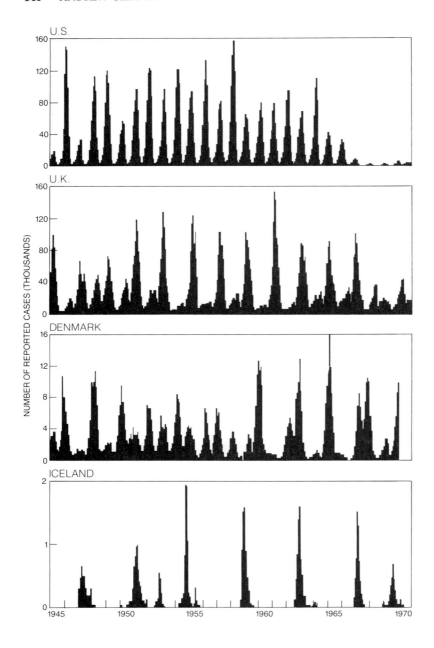

Figure 11.2 POPULATION SIZE strongly affects the pattern of measles epidemics. In the U.S., which had a population of 200 million in 1970, measles epidemics recurred annually until the mid-1960's, when a vaccination program began. Between epidemics measles was always present at a low level. In the U.K., with a population of 50 million in 1970, and Denmark, with a population of five million, there was a similar pattern except that the measles epidemics tended to come respectively at intervals of two and three years. In Iceland, with a population of 200,000 in 1970, the epidemics were less regular. Between epidemics there was a period averaging three years when the virus was not reported on the island.

to the epidemics of measles, significant outbreaks of influenza, typhoid fever and whooping cough.

Since 1896 the chief physician of Iceland has published a detailed annual account of public health called *Heilbrigdisskýrslur* (literally "Health Reports"). The account includes monthly reports of the number of cases of major diseases in each of the 50 medical districts of the island. In addition it includes narratives by local medical officers describing the course of the epidemics in their district. The narratives give details of the severity and pattern of spread of each epidemic, the external source of the disease (if the source was known) and how the virus was diffused from village to village or from farm to farm. Even more detailed accounts are available in manuscript in the national archives.

Thus *Heilbrigdisskýrslur* and the manuscripts in the national archives provide two significant types of information. The district statistics yield a picture of the intensity and duration of an epidemic wave. The medical officers' narratives make it possible to reconstruct in detail the spread of the disease between geographic areas.

The records show that from 1896 through 1975 there were 16 distinct waves of measles. The epidemics varied in size from wave 1 in 1904, which included 822 reported cases, to wave 6 in 1936–37, which included 8,408 reported cases. In most countries medical reporting has improved greatly over the decades, but in Iceland even the early measles records appear to be fairly accurate. The waves lasted on the average for 19 months, and (leaving aside the unusually small and localized wave of 1904) in a typical epidemic only five of the 50 medical districts escaped infection. Between the waves there were periods averaging three years when the island was free of the measles virus. The geographic spread of a typical epidemic is shown in Figure 11.4.

T he narratives in *Heilbrigdisskýrslur* show that in order for an isolated Icelandic farmstead to be attacked by measles the virus must be carried a considerable distance by one infected individual or, what is more probable, by a chain of infected individuals. The virus must be carried several hundred miles across the sea to an entry port, then to a town or village and finally to the farmstead.

The general mechanism whereby measles is spread through human contact has been known for more than a century. In most epidemics, however, and in particular those that come in densely populated urban areas, the pathways of transmission are obscured by the large numbers of infected people mixing with the susceptible population. In formulating hypotheses on the spread of infection in such areas it has generally been necessary to adopt the simplifying assumption that contact in a human community is a kind of churning process where the motions of an individual are random. The particular value of *Heilbrigdisskyrslur* is that the reports enable the epidemiologist to discard that simplifying assumption and replace it with the actual movements of people carrying the virus between settlements.

Examination of the official records shows that the main reservoir from which measles was brought to

Iceland is northern Europe. When the virus reaches the island, it can spread along several routes. Wave 1 of 1904, which was confined to the fishing villages and isolated farms of northwestern Iceland, provides an interesting example of the process of virus introduction and transmission (see Figure 11.5).

The statistical data for wave 1, the first wave to be recorded in *Heilbrigdisskýrslur*, are not complete. There are 822 cases in the published records, but 1,993 cases are noted in the manuscript reports in the national archives. Some 40 percent of the 1,993 cases came in August, the peak month of the epidemic. Most of the cases were in Isafjordur, the main town of the region, where the physician was so overwhelmed that he was not able to keep detailed records; hence the discrepancy between the official total of 822 and the probable total of about 2,000. Twenty-three deaths attributable to measles were reported.

The path of movement of the disease was carefully noted in the narrative: "The disease came from Norway in April to the whaling stations in Hesteyri and Isafjordur. In the first place it stopped and there were no further infections, but in the latter it spread because the doctor was not informed at an early date. It spread most rapidly after a confirmation ceremony at the village of Eyri on May 22, 1904." From Eyri the epidemic was transmitted throughout the western part of the island.

This short excerpt from the official record throws light on three factors that are of much significance in understanding the epidemiological history of measles in Iceland. The first factor is the crucial role of the index case, whose spatial mobility is necessary to start a measles outbreak. By index case is meant an infected individual who introduces the infectious agent into a population where the agent had died out. Figure 11.6 shows the routes of index cases that triggered various Iceland epidemics. In wave 1 of the 1904 epidemic the index cases were the crew of a Norwegian whaling ship; in other waves the index cases were fishermen. The second factor is the contribution of communal activity to the spread of the disease. Communal activities served to bring the susceptible population together in the critical period when the virus had recently been brought into the area. The confirmation held at Eyri on May 22, 1904, is an example of a gathering of the local populace after which the virus was rapidly transmitted. The outbreak in Isafjordur began with "an adolescent girl who had been con-

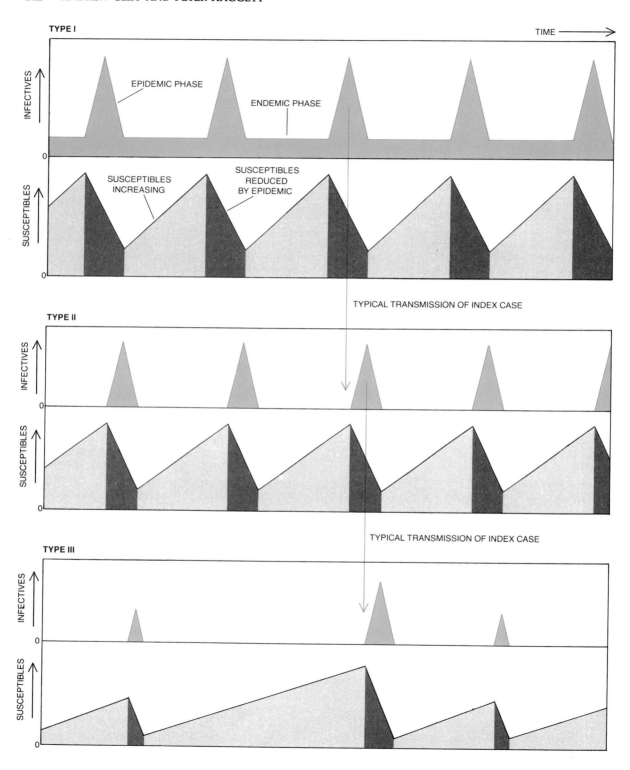

Figure 11.3 EPIDEMIC WAVES of measles can be divided into three types. In each panel the upper curve stands for the number of people in the community who are infected. The lower curve stands for the number who are susceptible to measles. Large communities show Type I waves (*top*). The virus is endemic: between epidemics there are always a few cases of measles. Medium-size communities show Type II waves (*middle*). These waves are regular but discontinuous; the population is too small to sustain the disease on an endemic basis. Between epidemics the virus dies out and is reintroduced from the large community during an epidemic there (*arrows*). Small communities show Type III waves (*bottom*). These waves are discontinuous and irregular.

firmed at Eyri and came from there to the town for domestic service."

The third factor that influenced how fast and how far the epidemic spread was the countermeasures implemented against it. The countermeasures generally took the form of interrupting contact between those who were infected and the rest of the people in the community: putting ships' crews in quarantine, putting measles patients in fever hospitals or isolating an infected farm household.

When the movement of the index cases and the resulting spread of the disease are traced in all 16 measles waves, it becomes clear that measles epidemics in Iceland tend to have three stages. In the first stage the virus is introduced to Reykjavik from outside Iceland, or is introduced from elsewhere in Iceland to Reykjavik soon after it arrives on the island. In the second stage the infection spreads from the capital to the provincial urban centers: Isafjordur in the northwest, Akureyri in the north and Egilsstadir and Seydisfjordur in the east. At the same time the virus diffuses out from Reykjavik into the region in southwestern Iceland surrounding the capital. In the third stage the disease spreads from the regional centers into their hinterland and begins to reach the outlying farms and fishing villages.

The account in *Heilbrigdisskýrslur* of the progress of the 16 waves of measles through the medical districts can also be utilized in a quantitative way to measure the time taken by the virus to reach a particular area. Such measurements confirm the qualitative three-stage model. The official record shows that Reykjavik is reached on the average within 1.5 months of the time the virus arrives on the island. The figures for the regional centers are as follows: Isafjordur 6.5 months, Akureyri from five

to eight months, Egilsstadir five months and Seydisfjordur 9.3 months. The only small towns and villages reached before the provincial centers are those near the capital. The isolated parts of northwestern Iceland are generally not reached until from 12 to 18 months after the start of the outbreak in Reykjavik.

Another chronological pattern that is of interest is the seasonal trend in the diffusion of the disease. If the movements of the index cases in the 16 waves are classified according to the month in which the disease was transmitted, it becomes evident that the spread of the disease has seasonal peaks and dips. In northern temperate climates measles, like many other infectious diseases of childhood, most frequently spreads in the winter. In Iceland, on the other hand, over much of the period since 1896 the transmission of measles has shown two peaks: until 1946 there was a peak in May and June in addition to the winter maximum. The local medical officers offer two reasons for the island's having a summer peak. One reason is that human mobility, which was severely limited by the subarctic winters, increased after the spring thaw. The other is that the major communal activity of haymaking began in June.

Tracing the movements of the index cases around the island can yield much information about the geographic and chronological patterns of measles waves. In order to apply the categories derived from Bartlett and Black, however, a count must be made of measles cases in each community over a period of time. When the number of cases and their timing are noted, it is found that since 1945 Iceland as a whole has shown the Type II pattern: the waves were fairly regular but between epidemics the measles virus apparently disappeared from the island. From 1896 through 1945, on the other hand, the pattern on the island seems to have been that of Type III.

If the number of cases in the individual communities is examined, a more complex pattern emerges. The largest communities have shown a consistent Type II pattern throughout the 20th century. This includes Reykjavik and its hinterland and the four outlying cities of Isafjordur, Akureyri, Egilsstadir and Seydisfjordur. The small towns and villages other than those in the neighborhood of the capital, however, showed waves of Type III.

The small communities vary in the number of epidemics they escaped. Half of the 16 waves failed

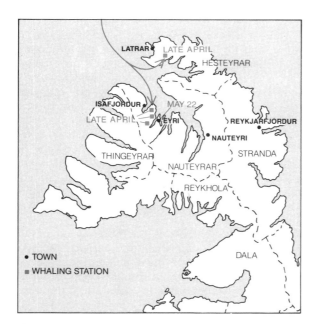

Figure 11.4 MEASLES EPIDEMIC in Iceland from November, 1946, through June, 1947. Blue circles stand for medical districts where one or two cases were reported; green, three to 20 cases; orange, 21 to 200 cases; red, 201 or more cases. Open circles are districts where no cases were reported but where cases had been reported the previous month. In the first stage cases appear in the capital city, Reykjavik (1). In the second stage measles were carried to the cities of Akureyri, Isafjordur and Egilsstadir and to the area surrounding Reykjavik (2–4). In the third stage the disease spread around the regional urban centers and reached the remote communities (5–8).

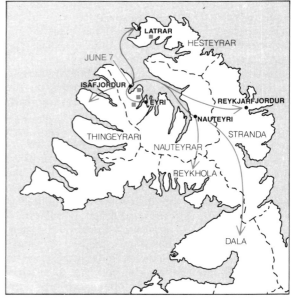

Figure 11.5 MEASLES EPIDEMIC OF 1904 was largely confined to the sparsely populated northwest peninsula of Iceland. The lines on the map show the routes of the spread of the disease. The virus was brought to Iceland in late April by the crew of a Norwegian whaling ship (left). Measles appeared first in a group of whaling stations. At a confirmation service at the nearby village of Eyri on May 22 many residents of the area were exposed to the measles virus. From there the infection was carried to Isafjordur, the largest city in the area, in early June (right). From Isafjordur the measles virus was dispersed throughout the entire peninsula during the summer months.

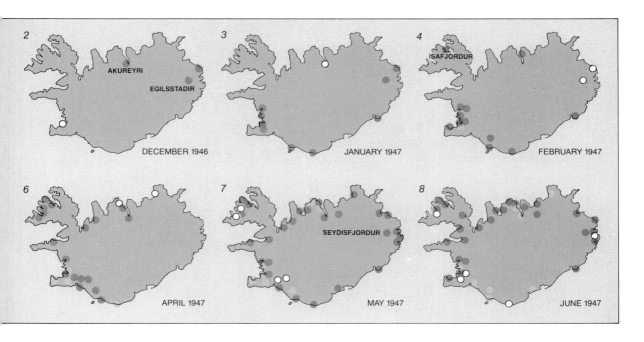

to reach the offshore island of Flatey. Substantial parts of the northwestern peninsula and of the north coast, which are sparsely populated and remote, missed two or more of the 16. As a rule medical districts with a population of 2,000 or more were reached by all the waves. If a district had a population of fewer than 2,000, its chance of missing a particular epidemic depended on how remote from the urban centers it was.

One of the fundamental goals of epidemiology has long been to formulate testable theories that could serve to project the course of future epidemics. Most of the attempts to devise such theories have had a simple basic structure. The number of people who will be infected in an epidemic wave is derived from the mixing of those who are susceptible with those who are already infected. These relations are expressed in a set of equations where the rate of mixing of the groups is controlled by factors termed diffusion constants. When such equations are calibrated to take account of the clinical history of the disease, the local vaccination rate and the recovery rate, they can generate a fairly good approximation of an epidemic wave train.

Knowledge of the geographic pattern of contact can be utilized to calibrate such equations on geographic principles as well as medical ones and thereby make the general theory more specific (see Figure 11.7). A single set of equations for the country as a whole can be replaced by a separate set for each medical district. The equations for a district include a diffusion constant that expresses the intensity of contact in the district rather than a generalized constant for the larger area.

Each set of equations is in essence a mathematical portrait of the factors that influence the course of the epidemic in a particular district. Having constructed such a portrait for each medical district, the sets of equations can be linked. The linkage depicts the exchange of infected and susceptible people between adjacent districts. What is meant by adjacent, of course, depends on maps of the movements of the index cases rather than on a map of linear distances. For example, in epidemiological terms Reykjavik can be regarded as a near neighbor of every other Icelandic community no matter how distant the other community is on a straight line.

The results obtained so far suggest that forecasting epidemics is likely to prove as difficult as forecasting snowfall. In both cases there are dangers in

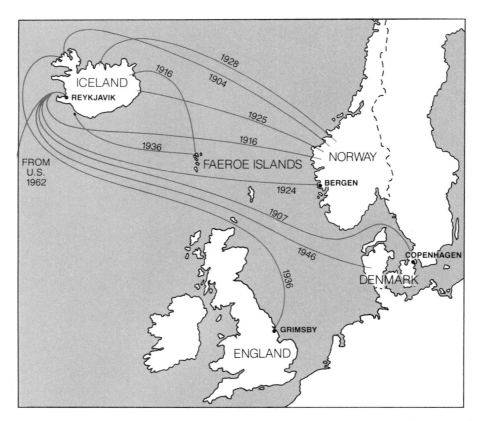

Figure 11.6 INDEX CASE is an infected individual who introduces measles into a population where the virus had died out. The map shows the routes that were taken to Iceland by the index cases who began measles epidemics on the island (where the route is known) from 1896 to 1975.

forecasting what does not happen as well as in failing to forecast what does. What is clear from the experiments in Iceland is that if more reliable models are to be constructed, it is necessary to understand the geographic pattern of the disease. Estimates incorporating geographic elements are consistently more accurate than those in which spatial elements are ignored.

Although the geographic pattern of the diffusion of measles in Iceland has been quite stable since 1900, the chronological pattern of the measles waves has changed considerably since World War II. The changes in the chronological form of the waves appear to be the result of the process of modernization, which has linked Iceland to the rest of the world and brought Icelandic settlements closer to one another. As a result the island's unusual seasonal pattern, with its winter and summer

peaks, has been eliminated. The summer peak has gradually disappeared, and Iceland currently has the single winter peak found in the northern temperate countries.

The second development has been a sharp change in the shape and timing of the epidemic waves. Before 1945 the measles waves varied greatly in amplitude. In addition the epidemics were separated by intervals that were often irregular and could be quite long. Since World War II the waves have tended to be more regular in amplitude and to be separated by shorter and more uniform intervals (see Figure 11.8).

The reason for the change is that the intensity of contact with the virus reservoirs of Europe and the U.S. has greatly increased. When most travel was by sea, the diffusion of the virus from mainland reservoirs to the island was occasional and irregular. The

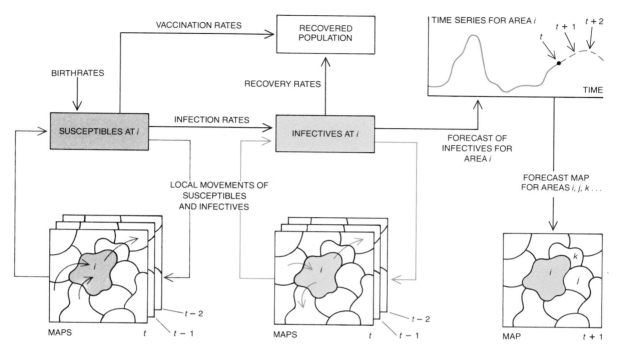

Figure 11.7 EPIDEMIC FORECAST is a prediction of how measles might spread in the immediate future. The forecast is based on a number of factors that are shown schematically for area *i* at time *t*. Each arrow corresponds to an equation. The susceptible population of the district is determined by the birthrate, the vaccination rate and the movement of susceptible people into and out of the district. The infected population is determined by the infection rate and the recovery rate. Combining these factors yields an estimate of the level of measles in area *i* at time *t* + 1. Linking the equations for all the medical districts yields the pattern of the epidemic across Iceland at time *t* + 1.

conversion of Keflavik Airport near the capital into a major staging post for international air travel, however, has led to the island's being at continuous risk of infection carried by air travelers. In the 30 years from 1945 to 1975 air-passenger traffic to Iceland increased by a factor of 15. As a result of the increase in exposure, whenever the susceptible population in Iceland reaches the minimum necessary for an epidemic, there is the risk of a measles wave diffusing out from Reykjavik.

As Iceland has become more closely bound to northern Europe and the U.S. the outlying areas of the island have acquired closer bonds to the capital. The epidemiology of the hinterland now closely resembles that of Reykjavik. Before World War II there was a notable difference between the epidemic waves in the capital and those in other places. The waves in Reykjavik were faster and more intense than the waves elsewhere: they had a shorter time to the infection peak, a shorter duration and a greater amplitude.

Since 1945, however, the two patterns have converged. The speed, duration and intensity of the epidemic waves in the hinterlands are now about equal to those in the capital. The convergence has resulted both from a decrease in the velocity of the waves in Reykjavik and an increase in velocity in the rest of the country. The slowing of the waves in Reykjavik results partly from improvements in health care there. From 1916 through 1972 the number of physicians per 1,000 people in the capital rose from 1.0 to 2.6; the increase in the rest of Iceland was only from .7 to .8.

The velocity and the intensity of the waves outside Reykjavik have increased in part because of advances in transportation and communication. Since World War II a network of roads has been

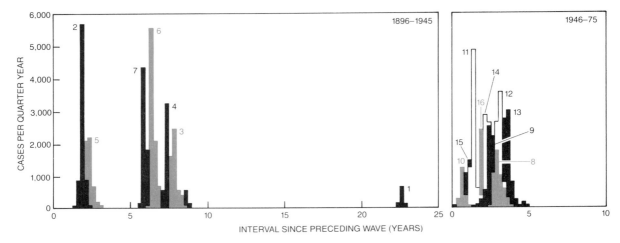

Figure 11.8 INTERVALS BETWEEN MEASLES WAVES have become shorter and more regular since 1945. The bars stand for the number of measles cases per quarter year in each of the 16 waves. The panel at the left is for the seven waves through 1945. The panel at the right is for the nine waves after 1945. The position of the bars on the horizontal axis indicates the interval since the preceding wave. Before 1946 the intervals were irregular and could be quite long; the longest interval was more than 20 years. Since 1946 the intervals have been short and regular, averaging about three years. In the same period the epidemic waves have also become somewhat more uniform in amplitude.

constructed around Iceland, which has reduced dependence on sea travel. Moreover, the island has the most frequently utilized domestic airline system in Europe, as measured by the number of passenger miles per year per 1,000 residents.

Sociological changes have accompanied the decreasing isolation of the villages and farms, and some of these changes have contributed to the changing character of the measles waves. For example, before 1945 the rural areas had an educational system in which a teacher visited outlying farms for a few weeks each term. Since the war this ambulatory system has largely been replaced by boarding schools where farm children spend weeks at a time. The vulnerable school-age population is therefore more concentrated and more accessible to the measles virus than it was in earlier decades.

The diffusion of measles in Iceland is not a static phenomenon but a dynamic process that reflects the transformation of the island's social structure. What lessons does the story hold for public-health workers who seek to eradicate the measles virus elsewhere in the world? The advances in transportation and communication in Iceland have made many communities that were once remote from Reykjavik adjacent to the capital in an epidemiolog-

ical sense. Such communities, which in the past had Type III measles waves, now have Type II waves.

Conquering the measles virus in the world as a whole depends on reversing this trend. Through the administration of measles vaccine large populations will begin to have the properties of smaller ones. In theory a global vaccination program could systematically reduce the size of susceptible populations to the level where the chain of infected people would not be maintained. In terms of the Bartlett model that would mean reducing the waves in all communities from Type I to Type II and from Type II to Type III.

In the U.S. the program coordinated by the Centers for Disease Control (CDC) brought a spectacular reduction in cases of measles (see the U.S. data in Figure 11.2). Other countries, notably Australia, are showing an interest in this program. Medical opinion is divided on the feasibility of eliminating measles at the global level: the costs and the logistic problems would certainly be many times greater than those encountered in the elimination of smallpox. Even if the global eradication of measles in this century remains a dream, more parts of the world could undoubtedly become almost free of the disease. A significant first step would be containing the virus in a decreasing number of reservoir areas of Type I.

Although that is an appealing vision, there is still a large gap between epidemiological theory and public-health practice. Furthermore, in populations that are partially vaccinated there is a risk of raising the average age of infection; adult measles infections are in some cases more serious than childhood ones. To avoid such hazards the distance between theory and practice must be diminished. Geographic reconstruction of the way diseases move through human populations can help to diminish that distance and help in the design of programs to contain infectious diseases. In this effort the islands of the world could well prove to be a uniquely valuable epidemiological laboratory.

POSTSCRIPT

Epidemics of infectious disease are often compared with forest fires. Once fire has spread through an area, it does not recur until new trees have grown up. Epidemics in humans develop when a large population of susceptible individuals is present. If most individuals are immune, then an epidemic will not occur. Epidemiologists often discuss the concept of herd immunity: If most of a population is immune, the rest of the population is protected because the probability of spread of the disease through the population is too low. For instance, only about 70 percent of the population in the United States is immune to polio, yet there is essentially no polio disease in the United States; immunized individuals are protecting those who, for economic or religious reasons, have not been immunized. For a highly infectious disease such as smallpox or measles, the proportion of immune individuals necessary to confer immunity is much higher, 90 to 95 percent.

Measles is an excellent disease for the study of epidemics, since it is of such widespread occurrence and its diagnosis is so easy. There are two kinds of measles, the conventional disease, sometimes called rubeola, and so-called German measles, generally called rubella. Both are caused by paramyxoviruses, but it is rubeola that has been responsible for massive epidemics.

Before the development of a successful vaccine, measles was one of the most common diseases of childhood. In developed countries such as the United States, death from measles has always been rare, but in developing countries, where childhood malnutrition is prevalent, measles is a severe disease with a fatality rate of 5 to 10 percent. Thus, even though measles has been virtually eradicated from most developed countries, an understanding of measles epidemics and their control is of great importance. Even in developed countries, measles often causes severe symptoms in adults.

Islands have often served as natural laboratories for epidemiologists. Iceland makes an especially suitable research site because its population is relatively uniform racially and its highly developed public-health bureaucracy has ensured that complete and accurate records are available. However, since World War II, Iceland is no longer an isolated location and the characteristic waves of measles that occurred earlier are no longer so easy to perceive. Thus, most of the epidemics described in the present article occurred before 1946.

The concept of an index case is an important one in epidemiology. The index case is the infected individual who, generally unwittingly, introduces the infectious agent into the population. Studies on the incidence of the common cold on the island of Spitzbergen, which is closed to shipping throughout the whole winter, have shown that it is the first boat in the spring that introduces the index case and triggers the next cold epidemic.

An especially tragic example of the importance of the index case was the introduction of tuberculosis into islands of the South Pacific by the English navigator Captain James Cook. By all accounts, tuberculosis was absent from the Polynesian populations before Captain Cook's visit. Although a relatively benign disease in Europeans, it spread through the native populations like an acute infection.

The Birth of the U.S. Biological-Warfare Program

Recently declassified government files reveal the events that led to research on biological weapons. Now a divisive public issue, the program started out as an obscure operation in World War II.

. . .

Barton J. Bernstein
June, 1987

"Why is it so confidential to destroy insect pests?" a perplexed Franklin D. Roosevelt asked his special assistant Wayne Coy on July 14, 1943, when the U.S. had been embroiled in World War II for a year and a half. The chief executive was looking over a Department of Agriculture request for $405,000 to support research on insect infestations and plant diseases. He knew only that his Bureau of the Budget was not informed about this project and that the War Department had instructed Agriculture to keep it secret.

Roosevelt asked Coy to investigate the mysterious enterprise. Two days later Coy told the president that details of the project were guarded for good reasons and suggested he ask a man named George W. Merck to tell him more about the work. Merck was in charge of a civilian adjunct to the War Department. Its mission was research on biological warfare.

Compared with the $2-billion Manhattan Project that gave rise to the atomic bomb, U.S. research on biological warfare during World War II was a small-scale venture: the project had a staff of about 4,000 workers, including scientists, and its total cost was about $60 million, including construction. Perhaps, then, it is not surprising that President Roosevelt did not remember that the Agriculture Department had joined the Army's Chemical Warfare Service in its efforts to develop biological weapons.

Neither Roosevelt nor Harry S. Truman, his successor, ever confronted the decision to order a biological attack. The issue of biological warfare did not end, however, with World War II. The U.S. continued to develop its biological arsenal for many years after the war and American interest in funding such research has recently revived: appropriations for biological-weapons projects, which hit rock bottom during the Nixon, Ford and Carter administrations, climbed back to $60 million last year.

In September, 1986 a multinational congress met to review a 1972 convention that bans the development, production and possession of biological weapons, including toxins, for offensive purposes. Both the U.S. and the U.S.S.R. are signatories of the convention, but the U.S. has charged the Soviets with several violations. Following up on informal contacts, scientific contingents from both countries gathered at Geneva in April, 1987 to try to hammer out mutually acceptable measures for treaty verification. Given the controversial American allegations, Soviet reluctance at disclosure and disputes on each side about the other's activity, the 1972 agreement could be in trouble.

Under these circumstances it may be instructive to study the origins of the program and examine the decisions that stayed the use of biological weapons by the U.S. in World War II. About 100 key documents have helped me to piece together an account of the wartime deliberations. The documents were culled from thousands of American papers declassified on special request and from British files that were once secret.

In World War I chemical agents such as chlorine and mustard gas killed or injured more than a million soldiers and civilians. Outrage at these deaths prompted 40 nations in 1925 to sign the Geneva Protocol, which prohibited the first use of chemical and biological weapons but placed no constraints on research, production and stockpiling. In subsequent years most major industrial powers maintained active development programs. Although the U.S. signed the Geneva Protocol, it did not ratify the treaty until 1975.

The U.S. Army started conducting biological-warfare research in 1941 through its Chemical War-

fare Service, but American efforts did not become substantial until 1942. In February of that year a special committee appointed by the National Academy of Sciences submitted a report to Secretary of War Henry L. Stimson containing recommendations for the future of the biological-warfare program (see Figure 12.1). Stimson had requested the report a few months before the bombing of Pearl Harbor.

The committee, composed of eminent biologists such as Edwin B. Fred of the University of Wisconsin and Stanhope Bayne-Jones of Yale University, concluded that an enemy attacking with biological weapons could gravely harm human beings, crops and livestock. Although the report stressed defense and called for work on vaccines and protection of the water supply, the committee also recommended, rather vaguely, that the U.S. conduct research on the offensive potential of bacterial weapons.

Spurred by the scientists' warnings, Stimson sought presidential approval for a formal biological-warfare program that would include a small group of advisers to coordinate and direct all government research. "We must be prepared," Stimson wrote to Roosevelt in an April 1942 memorandum. "And the matter must be handled with great secrecy as well as great vigor."

Stimson never mentioned that the Chemical Warfare Service had already begun research into biological weaponry, and the president probably did not know of the program. Still, the chemical service later received millions of dollars in appropriations

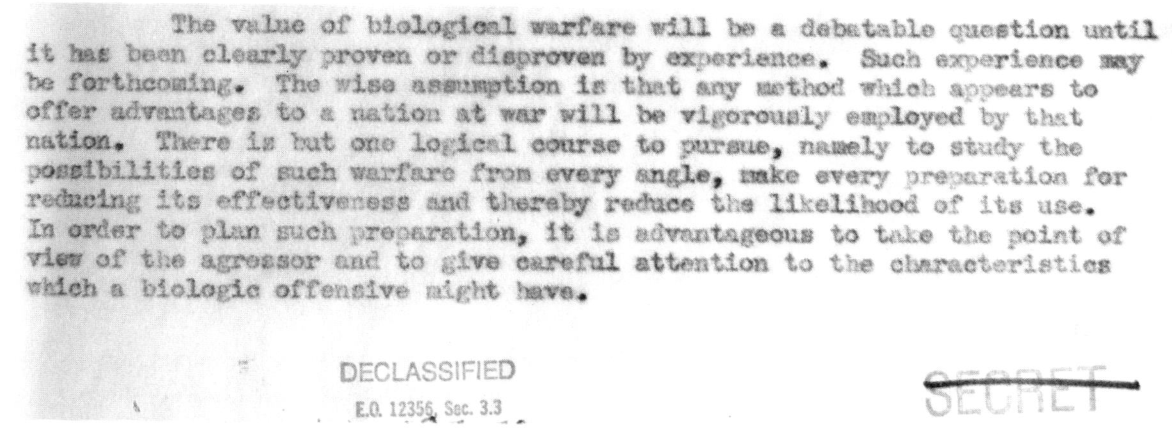

The value of biological warfare will be a debatable question until it has been clearly proven or disproven by experience. Such experience may be forthcoming. The wise assumption is that any method which appears to offer advantages to a nation at war will be vigorously employed by that nation. There is but one logical course to pursue, namely to study the possibilities of such warfare from every angle, make every preparation for reducing its effectiveness and thereby reduce the likelihood of its use. In order to plan such preparation, it is advantageous to take the point of view of the agressor and to give careful attention to the characteristics which a biologic offensive might have.

DECLASSIFIED
E.O. 12356, Sec. 3.3

SECRET

Figure 12.1 EXCERPT FROM RECOMMENDATIONS made in a 1942 National Academy of Sciences report stresses the feasibility of conducting research on biological weapons. The report probably persuaded President Roosevelt to create the War Research Service.

through the Army's budget and became more instrumental in the biological-warfare program than the small advisory group that directed it. Why did Stimson press for the group?

Perhaps it was because, as he told Roosevelt, "biological warfare is dirty business." Stimson hoped to legitimize the research at the Chemical Warfare Service by naming civilians as monitors. Whereas some members of the National Academy of Sciences committee thought the program should be administered by the War Department, top Army officials preferred the establishment of a civilian agency with ties to the armed services. Stimson explained their reasoning to Roosevelt: "Entrusting the matter to a civilian agency would help in preventing the public from being unduly exercised over any ideas that the War Department might be contemplating the use of this weapon offensively."

Stimson suggested hiding the "germ warfare" advisory group in a New Deal welfare agency, called the Federal Security Agency, that oversaw the Public Health Service and Social Security. He wanted an academic luminary to direct the program, someone familiar with the university research system and skilled in administration. After a cabinet meeting on May 15 Roosevelt admitted he had not yet read the secretary's plan but told him to go ahead with it anyway. A week later Stimson discussed his ideas with Secretary of Agriculture Claude R. Wickard, whose agency would later take part in the research coordinated by the advisory group, and with Paul V. McNutt, who led the Federal Security Agency.

By midsummer three candidates had rejected an offer to head the new group: economist Walter W. Stewart, who chaired the Rockefeller Foundation; geographer Isaiah Bowman, president of Johns Hopkins University; and economist Edmund Ezra Day, president of Cornell University. Finally, in August, chemist George W. Merck, president of the pharmaceutical firm Merck & Co., Inc., accepted the position (see Figure 12.2).

The innocuously named War Research Service (WRS) started out in mid-1942 with an initial allocation of $200,000. Wide contacts among major biologists and physicians enabled the eight-member directorate to initiate secret work in about 28 American universities, including Harvard University, Columbia University, Cornell University, the University of Chicago, Northwestern University, Ohio State University, the University of Notre Dame, the University of Wisconsin, Stanford University and the University of California. By January of 1943 the WRS had contracted with William A. Hagan of Cornell to explore offensive uses of botulism and with J. Howard Mueller of the Harvard Medical School to study anthrax.

Anthrax and botulism remained the foci of biological-warfare research during the war. Both deadly diseases are of bacterial origin, and the bacteria are hardy and prolific. Both have very short incubation periods, lasting for only a few days or even hours. The tough but virulent anthrax spores can be inhaled or absorbed through breaks in the skin; botulism results from ingestion of the bacterial poison botulin.

Reaching beyond college campuses, the WRS empowered the Chemical Warfare Service to expand greatly its own work on biological warfare. In 1942 and 1943 the chemical service received millions of dollars to build research facilities. The most notable one was Camp Detrick in Frederick, Md. (now Fort Detrick), which cost nearly $13 million. The service also hired many scientists to work there and elsewhere in the newly enlarged system.

The scientists, drawn largely from university faculties, put aside their repugnance at developing agents of death because the work seemed necessary in the exceptional situation of World War II (see Figure 12.3). Theodor Rosebury, a Columbia microbiologist, argued in early 1942 that "the likelihood that bacterial warfare will be used against us will surely be increased if an enemy suspects that we are unprepared to meet it and return blow for blow." Soon afterward Rosebury entered the Chemical Warfare Service's laboratory and became a leader at Camp Detrick. "We were fighting a fire [the Axis]," he later wrote, "and it seemed necessary to risk getting dirty as well as burnt."

Stimson and McNutt might well have applauded these sentiments, but they would have been astonished at Rosebury's view of who held the reins. Rosebury believed the ethical concerns of the scientists in his laboratory governed the use of the weapons they were creating. He wrote years later: "Civilians, in or out of uniform, made all the important decisions; the professional military kept out of the way. We resolved the ethical question just as other equally good men resolved the same question at Oak Ridge and Hanford and Chicago and Los Alamos."

History tells a different story. Even though the

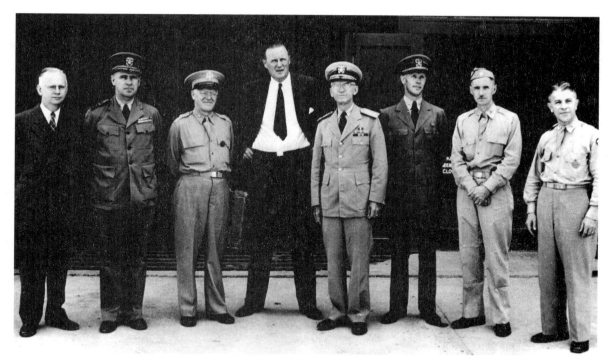

Figure 12.2 ADVISERS FOR BIOLOGICAL WEAPONS gathered at Camp Detrick to consult technical experts. George W. Merck, president of Merck & Co., Inc., is in the middle. Other advisers, from the left, are scientific director Ira L. Baldwin, Capt. Nathaniel S. Prime, Brig. Gen. W. A. Borden, Rear Adm. Julius Zurer, Comdr. William B. Sarles, Colonel Woolpert and Lt. Col. Norman Pyle. Baldwin and Sarles were on temporary loan from the University of Wisconsin-Madison.

president himself may not have set the course of the WRS, it seems clear that the key decisions were made in Washington, not in the laboratory.

In spite of Paul McNutt's primary concern with welfare and social services, he kept an eye on the secret biological-warfare program hidden in his agency. In February of 1943 McNutt informed President Roosevelt that the last of the WRS's $200,000 was being spent. The president, he said, would have to decide whether to "go more deeply into two or three . . . projects now under way." By April, with Stimson's approval, McNutt requested another $25,000 for the WRS fiscal 1943 budget and a total of $350,000 for fiscal 1944. Two days later Roosevelt endorsed McNutt's request with one laconic notation: "O.K. F.D.R." The WRS 1944 budget grew again several months later, when Roosevelt expanded it to $460,000.

In keeping with the tight security of the program, McNutt did not commit particular projects or details to writing, even in his correspondence with the president. Roosevelt's own files contain fewer than a dozen letters and memorandums on biological warfare. Of the handful pertaining to 1942 and 1943, most deal with the small appropriations and administrative arrangements for the War Research Service. Perhaps in discussions with McNutt and Stimson or in meetings with Gen. George C. Marshall, the trusted Army chief of Staff, Roosevelt was kept informed of the additional millions of dollars in appropriations going to the biological-warfare work of the Chemical Warfare Service. Not one of the available records, however, shows that Roosevelt was receiving such reports.

Meanwhile the chemical service was enlarging its facilities for development, testing and production. In addition to the 500-acre Camp Detrick site, a

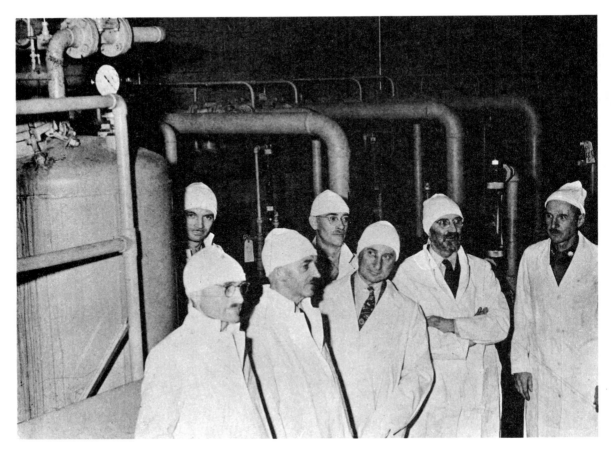

Figure 12.3 TEAM OF SCIENTISTS inspects the facilities at Camp Detrick. In 1943 the camp was the center of the Chemical Warfare Service's biological-weapons program. Pictured are (*front, from left*) Paul Hudson of Ohio State University, Guilford B. Reed of Queen's University, Charles A. Mitchell of the Dominion Department of Agri-culture, Everitt G. D. Murray of McGill University and Col. Oram C. Woolpert; behind them are James Craigie (*right*) of the University of Toronto and Col. Arvo T. Thompson.

2,000-acre installation for field trials was established on Horn Island in Pascagoula, Miss. A 250-square-mile site near the Dugway Proving Ground in Utah was designated for bombing tests and 6,100 acres were secured for a manufacturing plant to be built near Terre Haute, Ind.

The technology was also advancing. With British technical assistance, the chemical service gained considerable ground in making biological bombs and in late 1943 began work on 500-pound anthrax bombs (see Figure 12.4). These bombs held 106 four-pound "bomblets" that would disperse and break on impact. The bombs were untested, but it was known that pulmonary anthrax, which causes lesions on the lungs, was almost invariably fatal.

The chemical service also succeeded in producing botulin, one of the most potent of all gastrointestinal poisons. Merely tasting food infected with the toxin is usually sufficient to cause severe illness or death. In natural outbreaks the death rate ranges from 16 to 82 percent, but by varying the toxin and the delivery mechanism, the scientists at Camp Detrick hoped to produce a reliably lethal weapon.

Bolstered by its progress, the Chemical Warfare Service began lobbying early in 1944 for an

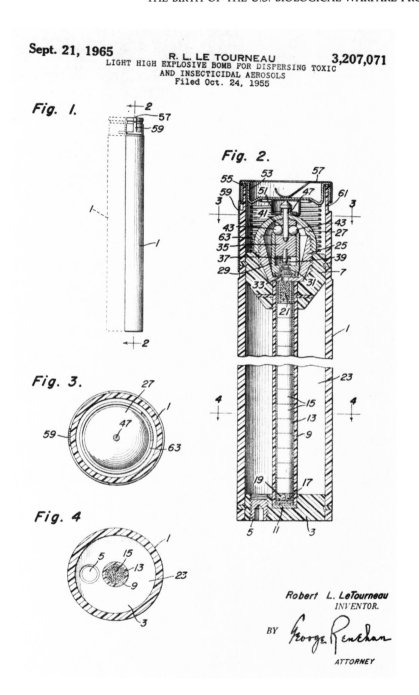

Sept. 21, 1965   R. L. LE TOURNEAU   3,207,071
LIGHT HIGH EXPLOSIVE BOMB FOR DISPERSING TOXIC
AND INSECTICIDAL AEROSOLS
Filed Oct. 24, 1955

Robert L. LeTourneau
INVENTOR.

BY George Renehan

ATTORNEY

Figure 12.4 PATENT ILLUSTRATION accompanying a 1955 filing by Robert L. Le Tourneau shows an "explosive bomb for dispersing toxic and insecticidal aerosols." The design may be a descendant of those proposed for anthrax bombs during World War II, when Le Tourneau was involved in biological-warfare research. Details of the anthrax bomb are still secret.

additional $2.5 million to finance the manufacture of anthrax and botulin bombs. The service could produce either 275,000 botulin bombs or one million anthrax bombs every month with that allocation, but it would need time to build factories. Hence the weapons would not be available in quantity until 1945, by which time, military strategists predicted, only the war with Japan would remain.

The service got its funds. Although the vision of a biological arsenal with which to confront the Japanese was tempting, a more urgent threat may have underscored the significance of the service's research. Early in 1944 Allied intelligence experts were beginning to fear that Germany's powerful new V-1 "buzz bombs" might soon be directed against Britain or the troops in Normandy, and that the missiles' warheads might be loaded with germ-warfare agents. The German high command, the experts warned, was facing a strategic crisis; it was assembling all its resources and might resort to biological warfare to gain a permanent advantage.

The analyses were based on so-called worst-case assumptions. They were not comforting; by June, 1944, the U.S. had probably prepared only a few anthrax bombs for testing, if any. Certainly no bombs were available for use against an enemy.

To deter Germany from launching a biological strike, military leaders arranged to inoculate about 100,000 soldiers against botulin, hoping to convince the Germans that Allied troops were preparing for biological retaliation. If Germany had actually staged a biological attack, Anglo-American forces would probably have retaliated with gas.

Germany never called the bluff. Hitler used only conventional explosives in the V-1. As a matter of fact, for reasons that are still not known he had barred all research on offensive biological warfare. The American program—deveoped substantially to deal with a German threat that never existed—remained untried.

W ork at Camp Detrick moved at a brisk pace. Many of the experiments were carried out in hastily constructed temporary buildings (see Figure 12.5). In May, 1944, Stimson and McNutt presented Roosevelt with a brief research summary that allotted only five lines to scientific developments. Much more could have been said. An anthrax plant received authorization through the Chemical Warfare Service to manufacture a million bombs and the service was making headway with short-range dispersal techniques for botulin in paste form. In November, Merck sent a report to Stimson and Marshall—but not to Roosevelt—that cryptically

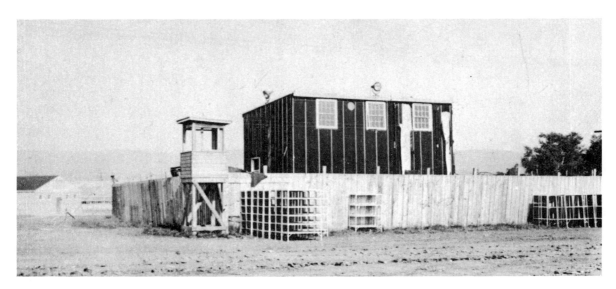

Figure 12.5 "BLACK MARIA," a somber tar-paper building, was constructed in 1944 to house biological-weapons experiments at Camp Detrick. A soldier armed with a sub-machine gun occupied the wood guard tower at the left. The building was razed soon after the war.

mentioned research on four additional "agents against men." Judging from other sources, these were probably brucellosis (undulant fever), psittacosis (parrot fever), tularemia (rabbit fever) and the respiratory disease glanders.

Merck said the Chemical Warfare Service was also developing "at least five agents for use against plants," (These agents are actually chemicals, but at the time they were defined as part of the biological program because they could kill crops.) A sixth compound, ammonium thiocyannate, was recommended for the decimation of "Japanese gardens."

These developments constituted 12 lines in Merck's short November report on biological warfare. The document is tucked away in Stimson's declassified Secretary of War records in Washington. There is no evidence that the secretary or the president devoted any attention to the scientific grist of the program.

Roosevelt neglected not only the science but also the politics of biological warfare. In spite of the considerable progress at Camp Detrick and fears of a German biological offensive, the president seems to have given the matter of biological warfare little thought. In 1942 and again in 1943 Roosevelt had promised publicly not to initiate gas warfare, but he threatened retaliation in kind if the Axis used gas. Apparently he never considered issuing a similar statement on germ warfare. Nor did any adviser propose such a warning to deter action by Germany or Japan.

In May, 1944, Roosevelt's ties to the biological-warfare program became even more tenuous when Stimson and McNutt urged him to abolish the War Research Service and make Merck a consultant to Stimson. The president readily acceded to this reorganization, which may have further distanced him from the secretive enterprise.

Then, in July, the president's military chief of staff Admiral William D. Leahy and several other advisers conducted in front of Roosevelt what Leahy later called "a spirited discussion of bacteriological warfare." The conversation focused on possible first use to destroy Japan's rice crop. Leahy wrote later that he recoiled from the idea; Roosevelt remained noncommittal. The president never indicated whether he would launch a biological-warfare attack in retaliation against Axis first use or whether he would countenance first use against Japan. (At the time claims were circulating that Japan had used biological warfare against China.) In stark contrast to his public pledges that the U.S. would not initiate gas warfare, Roosevelt thus bequeathed to Truman an ambiguous legacy regarding biological weapons.

Two weeks after Truman entered the White House in April of 1945, and a day after the president had received a lengthy briefing on the atomic bomb, Secretary Stimson got a memo from his special assistant Harvey H. Bundy. Bundy wrote that Merck and several other members of the biological-warfare program were proposing the use of chemicals against Japanese food crops. "It is a pretty serious step," the assistant cautioned, "and you may want to speak to the President." Stimson sent a note to Marshall asking to confer with him at his convenience.

From that point until the war's conclusion, emphasis on biological warfare shifted from bacteriological agents to crop defoliants. American scientists certified that the chemicals were not poisonous to humans; the Judge Advocate's Office concluded that their use would be legal because they were nontoxic to people and because the U.S., as a warring nation, "is entitled to deprive the enemy of food and water, and to destroy the sources of supply in his fields."

Stimson, although deeply troubled by the mass killing of noncombatants that American bombing had already caused, seemed prepared to accept the poisoning of Japanese crops. Given that General Marshall wanted to use gas against Japanese troops, he too was probably not unnerved by the tactic of crop poisoning. In May and June an Army Air Force general drew up an elaborate plan for destroying Japan's rice crops by dropping ammonium thiocyanate on rice-producing areas near six major cities: Tokyo, Yokohama, Osaka, Nagoya, Kyoto and Kobe. The commander of the Air Force, Gen. Henry H. Arnold, rejected the plan on tactical rather than moral grounds. Bombing Japan's industry and cities, he judged, would have "earlier and more certain impact."

When other military planners discussed the use of crop poison against Japan, they, like Arnold and his staff, gave primacy to tactical problems. Some questioned whether the supply of chemicals was sufficient; some thought the destruction of the 1945 rice crop would not have any effect until 1946. By then, they believed, the war would have been won and American occupation forces would have the added burden of feeding a hungry civilian population.

On August 3, three days before the bombing of Hiroshima, Arnold's deputy, Lt. Gen. Ira C. Eaker, asked for a comprehensive report on crop destruction by air, including the capabilities of the Air Force, the best chemicals available and the best techniques for their application. He got the report on August 10, the day after the Nagasaki bombing. Four days later the war in the Pacific ended.

The nation's secretly developed U.S. germ-warfare arsenal was not forgotten in the final months of the war. One high-ranking Army general had commented earlier in the program's history that the Administration might consider a policy of first use against Japan. Later, strategists discussing retaliation concluded that if Japan broke the Geneva Protocol and resorted to gas agents, the U.S. should be prepared to respond with both gas and germ weapons. Adm. Donald B. Duncan, a staff member of the Joint Chiefs of Staff, pointed out that in some situations bacteriological attacks might be more effective than gas.

American beliefs about the morality of biological warfare, however, were never put to the test in World War II. The ultimate decision to use biological weapons would have fallen to Truman; he probably would have relied on the counsel of General Marshall, whom he greatly admired, and of Secretary Stimson, whom he regarded as a moral man. Having sanctioned the use of atomic bombs on Japanese cities, these key advisers might not have taken exception to poisoning rice fields to compel Japan's surrender.

Germ warfare, with its specters of epidemic and invisible poison, might have been harder to endorse. Years later, however, Truman implied in a letter to an associate that if the war in the Pacific had dragged on past mid-August, he would have employed both bacteriological and chemical agents —that, in effect, the atomic bombing he had approved was so much worse.

The U.S. continued the development and stockpiling of biological weapons until 1969, when, in response to the antiwar sentiments of the Vietnam era, President Nixon vowed to halt the programs and destroy the stores. Three years later the U.S. and more than 100 other nations signed the Biological and Toxin Weapons Convention, and many agreed to ban biological warfare outright.

At the beginning of the 1980's the U.S. began to suspect that the Soviet Union had an active biological-warfare program. The U.S. expanded its own program in response. Suspicions were prompted in part by a 1979 outbreak of anthrax that may or may not have escaped from a facility in Sverdlovsk that the U.S. asserts is a weapons laboratory.

The so-called yellow rain said to have fallen in Laos and Kampuchea has also fueled suspicions. The U.S. government maintains it is a fungal toxin supplied by the Soviets to Vietnam, although some experts say it is only bee dung (see "Yellow Rain," by Thomas D. Seeley, Joan W. Nowicke, Matthew Meselson, Jeanne Guillemin and Pongthep Akratanakul; SCIENTIFIC AMERICAN, September, 1985).

The clandestine research that began in World War II has thus grown substantially to become an object worthy of international debate. How might peacetime decisions be made? If the past gives any indication, it is probable that the real decision makers are not in the laboratory. In World War II scientists provided the expertise to conceive and develop novel weapons, but historical evidence demonstrates that they lacked any authority to control deployment and use. Both wartime presidents, although decked with the formal authority of the commander-in-chief, knew very little about the biological arsenal over which they presided. Ironically, much of that arsenal had been developed primarily to deal with a country, namely Germany, that never intended to develop a capacity for offensive biological warfare.

American experience during World War II warns that weapons conceived for deterrence or retaliation may become attractive and may seem morally justifiable for offensive strikes. Once the war machine gears up for action, scientists may not be able to constrain use of the technology they have created, particularly in a conflict that is deemed a "just" war.

POSTSCRIPT

Although there are a few parallels between the Manhattan Project, which built the atomic bomb, and the War Research Service, which conducted research on biological warfare, the outcomes of these two World War II projects have been quite different. The explosion of the first atomic bomb changed human society for all time but biological warfare research has had much lesser consequences. Although there is some evidence that biological warfare has been used during the Vietnam war and in the Iraq-Iran conflict, these have been isolated incidents.

It is clear that the original motivation of U.S. research scientists to begin biological warfare research was defensive in nature. At no time did any of the scientists involved believe that they were working on agents of destruction. However, the work of scientists often falls out of their control, and once a procedure with military potential has been developed, there is always a possibility that it will be used offensively. Fortunately, since 1972, all research on biological weapons has been terminated and any stockpiles destroyed.

The United States was not the only nation to pursue biological warfare research during World War II. An extensive research program was also developed in Great Britain—the Microbiological Research Establishment at Porton, Salisbury. The British and United States shared data and personnel. The British also have the notoriety of having done an actual field test with a biological weapon. Sometime during World War II, the British released spores of the pathogenic bacterium *Bacillus anthracis*, the causal agent of anthrax, on Gruinard Island, a small, isolated island off the coast of Scotland. Studies showed that the agent remained viable in the soil for many years and the island remains uninhabited today. (Sheep were reintroduced on this island in 1987 to determine whether the infectious agent might have finally disappeared.)

Most of the infectious agents that have been considered for biological warfare are transmitted by the respiratory route. Among these are *Yersinia pestis*, the causal agent of plague (see Chapter 1, "The Bubonic Plague"), the fungus *Coccidioides immitis* and the rickettsial pathogen *Coxiella burnetii*. In addition, much research has been done with the botulinum toxin, produced by the bacterium *Clostridium botulinum* (an organism that causes a rare type of food poisoning). The botulinum toxin has the reputation of being the most poisonous substance known, able to cause death at vanishingly small doses. The mortality rate from botulinum poisoning is high, from 60 to 70 percent, meaning that the agent would be highly effective if it could be delivered to a target population. One disadvantage of botulinum toxin is that it decomposes relatively rapidly in air, so that its effects would not remain long in the environment. However, for certain types of military operations this short-lived character might be desirable, since it would mean that the attacking force could quickly move into the territory once the enemy force had been terminated.

One encouraging note: the Fort Detrick laboratory was converted in the early 1970's to a cancer research laboratory.

The Authors

The Editor

THOMAS D. BROCK is a professor of bacteriology at the University of Wisconsin-Madison. He received his Ph.D. from Ohio State University in 1952 and has been on the faculties of Case Western Reserve University, Indiana University and the University of Wisconsin. Brock also worked at the Upjohn Company and directed an extensive research program at Yellowstone National Park, which led to the discovery of numerous new organisms. He is the author of numerous works, including the widely used textbook *Biology of Microorganisms*. With his wife, Kathie, he operates Science Tech Publishers, which publishes textbooks and advanced monographs in various fields of contemporary bioscience.

COLIN McEVEDY ("The Bubonic Plague") is psychiatric consultant at St. Bernard's Hospital on the outskirts of London. He qualified as a doctor in 1955, after studying at the University of Oxford, where he received a doctorate in medicine in 1971. He worked at the Institute of Aviation Medicine while in the Royal Air Force and trained in psychiatry at Maudsley Hospital and Middlesex Hospital.

DAVID W. FRASER and **JOSEPH E. McDADE** ("Legionellosis") are respectively president of Swarthmore College and associate director for laboratory science at the Center for Infectious Disease of the Centers for Disease Control, which he joined in 1975. Fraser was graduated from Haverford College and received his M.D. from Harvard Medical School in 1969. He has worked at the Mayo Graduate School of Medicine in Rochester, Minn., and the University of Pennsylvania and joined the CDC in 1977. McDade received his Ph.D. in microbiology from the University of Delaware in 1967 and has worked at the U.S. Army Biological Center at Fort Detrick, Md., and the University of Maryland School of Medicine.

GAIL S. HABICHT, GREGORY BECK and **JORGE L. BENACH** ("Lyme Disease") are affiliated with the department of pathology at the State University of New York at Stony Brook. Habicht earned a Ph.D. from Stanford University in 1965 and held positions at Rockefeller University and the Scripps Clinic and Research Foundation before moving to Stony Brook in 1971. Beck received his B.S. from SUNY at Albany in 1982 and then worked at the Veterans Administration Medical Center in Northport, N.Y. Benach, a research scientist with the New York State Department of Health since 1971, also teaches at Stony Brook. He earned a B.S. (1966) and a Ph.D. (1971) from Rutgers University.

WILLIAM L. LANGER ("Immunization against Smallpox before Jenner") was Archibald Cary Coolidge Professor of History emeritus at Harvard University. He received his B.A. in 1915, M.A. in 1920 and Ph.D. in 1923, all from Harvard. He was editor of *An Encyclopedia of World History*, first published in 1940, and the series *The Rise of Modern Europe*.

DONALD A. HENDERSON ("The Eradication of Smallpox"), a graduate of Oberlin College, received his M.D. from the University of Rochester in 1954 and his M.P.H. from Johns Hopkins University in 1960. He worked in the Epidemic Intelligence Service of the Department of Health, Education and Welfare from 1961 to 1966, when he joined the World Health Organization in Geneva to organize an intensified smallpox eradication program.

ANTHONY ROBBINS and **PHYLLIS FREEMAN** ("Obstacles to Developing Vaccines for the Third World") began studying the obstacles to the development of new vaccines in 1984, while they were working for the U.S. Congress. Robbins is professor of public health at the Boston University School of Medicine. He received a bachelor's degree from Harvard College (1962), an M.D. from the Yale University School of Medicine (1966) and a Master's of Public Administration from Harvard University (1969). Freeman is associate professor and chairman of the Law Center of the College of Public and Community Service at the University of Massachusetts at Boston. She earned her law degree from Northeastern University in 1975.

RICHARD A. LERNER ("Synthetic Vaccines") is chairman of the molecular biology department at the Research Institute of the Scripps Clinic in La Jolla, Calif. He obtained his M.D. from Stanford University in 1964. He has been affiliated with the Scripps Clinic since 1965, except for 1968–70, which he spent at the Wistar Institute of Anatomy and Biology in Philadelphia.

MILTON J. FRIEDMAN and **WILLIAM TRAGER** ("The Biochemistry of Resistance to Malaria") began their collaboration at Rockefeller University, where Friedman did his graduate work and where Trager is professor and head of the department of parasitology. Friedman, who was an undergraduate at Reed College and the University of Washington, is an assistant research biologist at the Cancer Research Institute of the University of California at San Francisco. Trager has been on the faculty at Rockefeller since 1934, the year after he received his Ph.D. from Harvard University.

G. NIGEL GODSON ("Molecular Approaches to Malaria Vaccines") has been professor and chairman of the department of biochemistry at the New York University School of Medicine since 1980. He received a Ph.D. from the University of London in 1962 and did postdoctoral work at the California Institute of Technology and the Yale University School of Medicine. In 1969 he was appointed to the faculty at Yale.

JOHN E. DONELSON and **MERVYN J. TURNER** ("How the Trypanosome Changes Its Coat") are respectively professor of biochemistry at the University of Iowa and director of the biochemical-parasitology program at the Merck Sharp & Dohme Research Laboratory in Rahway, N.J. Donelson has a B.S. from Iowa State University and a Ph.D. in biochemistry from Cornell University. In 1974, after postdoctoral work at the University of Cambridge and Stanford University, he joined the faculty at the University of Iowa. Donelson is also a Burroughs-Wellcome scholar in molecular parasitology. Turner received a Ph.D. in organic chemistry from the University of Sheffield in 1970. He was a postdoctoral fellow at Harvard University (1971–74) and at Queen Victoria Hospital in London (1974–77). In 1977 he became a fellow at the Medical Research Council's Molteno Institute at Cambridge. He joined Merck Sharp and Dohme in 1985.

ANDREW CLIFF and **PETER HAGGETT** ("Island Epidemics") are geographers who have worked together since 1968 on the quantitative aspects of geography, in particular the problem of how cultural innovations, economic forms and diseases are transmitted spatially in human populations. Cliff was educated at King's College of the University of London, Northwestern University and the University of Bristol. His Ph.D. in geography was awarded by Bristol in 1969. In 1972 he joined the faculty of the University of Cambridge. Haggett is professor of urban and regional geography at Bristol. He was educated at Cambridge and taught there and at University College London before joining the Bristol faculty in 1966.

BARTON J. BERNSTEIN ("The Birth of the U.S. Biological-Warfare Program") is professor of history and Mellon Professor of Interdisciplinary Studies at Stanford University. He received his Ph.D. from Harvard University and taught for two years at Bennington College before going to Stanford in 1965. During World War II he worked on a project on the deterrence and morality of biological warfare. He has written *The Politics and Policies of the Truman Administration* (1971) and *The Atomic Bomb* (1976).

Bibliographies

1. The Bubonic Plague

Ziegler, Philip. 1970. *The Black Death.* Harper & Row, Inc.

Biraben, Jean-Noël. 1975. *Les hommes et la peste en France et dans les pays Européens et Mediterranéens.* Mouton et Cie.

Dols, Michael W. 1977. *The Black Death in the Middle East.* Princeton University Press.

2. Legionellosis

Chandler, Francis W., Martin D. Hicklin and John A. Blackman. 1977. Demonstration of the agent of Legionnaires' disease in tissue. *New England Journal of Medicine* 297 (December 1): 1218–1220.

Fraser, David W., Theodore F. Tsai, Walter Orenstein, William E. Parkin, H. James Beecham, Robert G. Sharrar, John Harris, George F. Mallison, Stanley M. Martin, Joseph E. McDade, Charles Shepard, Philip S. Brachman and the Field Investigation Team. 1977. Legionnaires' disease: Description of an epidemic of pneumonia. *New England Journal of Medicine* 297 (December 1): 1189–1197.

McDade, Joseph E., Charles Shepard, David W. Fraser, Theodore F. Tsai, Martha A. Redus, Walter R. Dowdle and the Laboratory Investigation Team. 1977. Legionnaires' disease: Isolation of a bacterium and demonstration of its role in other respiratory disease. *New England Journal of Medicine* 297 (December 1): 1197–1203.

Glick, Thomas H., Michael B. Gregg, Bernard Berman, George Mallison, Wallace W. Rhodes, Jr., and Ira Kassanoff. 1978. Pontiac fever: An epidemic of unknown etiology in a health department. I. Clinical and epidemiologic aspects. *American Journal of Epidemiology* 197 (February): 149–160.

3. Lyme Disease

Steere, Allen C., Stephen E. Malawista, David R. Snydman, Robert E. Shope, Warren A. Andiman, Martin R. Ross and Francis M. Steele. 1977. Lyme arthritis: An epidemic of oligoarticular arthritis in children and adults in three Connecticut communities. *Arthritis and Rheumatism* 20 (January-February): 7–17.

Burgdorfer, Willy, Alan G. Barbour, Stanley F. Hayes, Jorge L. Benach, Edgar Grunwald and Jeffrey P. Davis. 1982. Lyme disease: A tick-borne spirochetosis? *Science* 216 (June 18): 1317–1319.

Habicht, Gail S., Gregory Beck, Jorge L. Benach, James L. Coleman and Kimberly D. Leichtling. 1985. Lyme disease spirochetes induce human and murine interleuken-1 production. *Journal of Immunology* 134 (May): 3147–3154.

Beck, Gregory, Gail S. Habicht, Jorge L. Benach and James L. Coleman. 1985. Chemical and biologic characterization of a lipopolysaccharide extracted from the Lyme disease spirochete (*Borrelia burgdorferi*). *Journal of Infectious Diseases* 152 (July): 108–117.

4. Immunization against Smallpox before Jenner

Klebs, Arnold C. 1913. The historic evolution of variolation. *Johns Hopkins Hospital Bulletin* XXIV (March): 69–83.

Dixon, C. W. 1962. *Smallpox.* J. & A. Churchill Ltd.

Creighton, Charles. 1965. *A history of epidemics in Britain.* Frank Cass & Co. Ltd.

King, Lester S. 1971. *The medical world of the eighteenth century.* Robert E. Kreiger Publishing Co., Inc.

Zielonski, Jason S. 1972. Inoculation: Pro and con. *Journal of the History of Medicine* XXVII (October): 447.

5. The Eradication of Smallpox

Dixon, C. W. 1962. *Smallpox.* J. & A. Churchill Ltd.

Henderson, Donald A. 1973. Smallpox. In *Maxcy-Rosenau preventive medicine and public health, 10th ed.,* ed. Philip E. Sartwell. Appleton-Century-Crofts.

Foege, William H., J. D. Millar and D. A. Henderson. 1975. Smallpox eradication in west and central Africa. *Bulletin of the World Health Organization* 52:209–222.

6. Obstacles to Developing Vaccines for the Third World

Committee on Issues and Priorities for New Vaccine Development, Institute of Medicine. 1986. *New vaccine development, Establishing priorities, Vol. 2: Diseases of importance in developing countries.* National Academy Press.

Warren, Kenneth S. 1986. New scientific opportunities and old obstacles in vaccine development. *Proceedings of the National Academy of Sciences* 83 (December): 9275–9277.

Walsh, Julia. 1988. *Establishing health priorities in the developing world.* United Nations Development Program. Adams Publishing Group.

Grant, James P. 1988. *The state of the world's children.* United Nations Children's Fund. Oxford University Press.

Plotkin, Stanley A., and Edward A. Mortimer. 1988. *Vaccines.* W. B. Saunders Co.

7. Synthetic Vaccines

Sutcliffe, J. G., T. M. Shinnick, N. Green, F.-T. Lie, H. L. Niman and R. A. Lerner. 1980. Chemical synthesis of a polypeptide predicted from nucleotide sequence allows detection of a new retroviral gene product. *Nature* 287 (October 30): 801–805.

Lerner, Richard A., J. Gregor Sutcliffe and Thomas M. Shinnick. 1981. Antibodies to chemically synthesized peptides predicted from DNA sequences as probes of gene expression. *Cell* 23 (February): 309–310.

Lerner, Richard A. 1982. Tapping the immunological repertoire to produce antibodies of predetermined specificity. *Nature* 299 (October 14): 592–596.

8. The Biochemistry of Resistance to Malaria

Armelagos, George J., and John R. Dewey. 1970. Evolutionary response to human infectious diseases. *Bioscience* 20 (March 1): 271–275.

Livingstone, Frank B. 1971. Malaria and human polymorphisms. *Annual Review of Genetics* 5:33–64.

Trager, William, and James B. Jensen. 1978. Cultivation of malarial parasites. *Nature* 273 (June 22): 621–622.

Luzzatto, L. 1979. Genetics of red cells and susceptibility to malaria. *Blood* 54 (October): 961–976.

9. Molecular Approaches to Malaria Vaccines

Nussenzweig, Ruth S. 1982. Progress in malaria vaccine development: Characterization of protective antigens. *Scandinavian Journal of Infectious Diseases,* Supplementum 36:40–45.

Godson, G. N., J. Ellis, P. Svec, D. H. Schlesinger and V. Nussenzweig. 1983. Identification and chemical synthesis of a tandemly repeated immunogenic region of *Plasmodium knowlesi* circumsporozoite protein. *Nature* 305 (September 1): 29–33.

Coppel, Ross L., Alan F. Cowman, Klaus R. Lingelbach, Graham V. Brown, Robert B. Saint, David J. Kemp and Robin F. Anders. 1983. Isolate-specific S-antigen of *Plasmodium falciparum* contains a repeated sequence of eleven amino acids. *Nature* 306 (December 22): 751–756.

Dame, John B., Jackie L. Williams, Thomas F. McCutchan, James L. Weber, Robert A. Wirtz, Wayne T. Hockmeyer, W. Lee Maloy, J. David Haynes, Imogene Schneider, Donald Roberts, Greg S. Sanders, E. Premkumar Reddy, Carter L. Diggs and Louis H. Miller. 1984. Structure of the gene encoding the immunodominant surface antigen on the sporozoite of the human malaria parasite *Plasmodium falciparum. Science* 225 (August 10): 593–599.

10. How the Trypanosome Changes Its Coat

Desowitz, Robert S. 1981. New Guinea tapeworms and Jewish grandmothers: Tales of parasites and people. In *The fly that would be king.* W. W. Norton and Co.

Turner, M. J. 1982. Biochemistry of the variant surface glycoproteins of salivarian trypanosomes. *Advances in Parasitology* 21:69–153.

Ransford, Oliver. 1983. *Bid the sickness cease—disease in the history of black Africa.* John Murray, Ltd.

Freymann, D. M., P. Metcalf, M. Turner and D. C. Wiley. 1984. Å-resolution X-ray structure of a variable surface glycoprotein from *Trypanosoma brucei. Nature* 311 (September 13): 167–169.

11. Island Epidemics

Bartlett, M. S. 1957. Measles periodicity and community size. *Journal of the Royal Statistical Society,* Series A, 120:48–70.

Black, Francis L. 1966. Measles endemicity in insular populations: Critical community size and its evolutionary implication. *Journal of Theoretical Biology* 11 (July): 207–211.

Cliff, A. D., P. Haggett, J. K. Ord and G. R. Versey. 1981. *Spatial diffusion: An historical geography of epidemics in an island community.* Cambridge University Press.

12. The Birth of the U.S. Biological-Warfare Program.

Brophy, Leo P., Wyndham D. Miles and Rexmond C. Cochrane. 1959. *The Chemical Warfare Service from laboratory to field.* U.S. Government Printing Office.

Bernstein, Barton J. 1987. Churchill's secret biological weapons. *Bulletin of the Atomic Scientists* 43 (January/February): 46–50.

Wright, Susan. 1987. New designs for biological weapons. *Bulletin of the Atomic Scientists* 43 (January/February): 43–46.

Harris, Elisa D. 1987. Sverdlovsk and yellow rain: Two cases of Soviet noncompliance. *International Security* 11 (Spring): 41–95.

Sources of the Photographs

1. Scala/Art Resource: Figure 1.2
   The Granger Collection: Figure 1.3

2. Joseph E. McDade, U.S. Centers for Disease Control, U.S. Public Health Service: Figure 2.3 (left)
   William W. Cherry, U.S. Centers for Disease Control: Figure 2.3 (right)
   Francis W. Chandler, U.S. Centers for Disease Control: Figure 2.6

3. Stanley F. Hayes, Willy Burgdorfer and M. D. Corwin, Rocky Mountain Laboratories: Figure 3.2
   Samuel L. Howard: Figure 3.5
   New York State Department of Health: Figure 3.6

4. World Health Organization: Figure 4.1
   Burndy Library: Figure 4.2
   National Library of Medicine: Figures 4.3 and 4.5
   Yale Medical Library, Clements C. Fry Collection: Figure 4.4

5. World Health Organization: Figures 5.1, 5.4 and 5.8
   Fritz Goro: Figure 5.6

6. U.S. Centers for Disease Control: Figure 6.3

Sean Sprague, United Nations Children's Fund: Figure 6.4

7. Arthur J. Olson, Research Institute of Scripps Clinic: Figures 7.3, 7.4, 7.6, 7.7 and 7.8

8. James B. Jensen: Figure 8.6
   William Trager: Figure 8.8

9. G. Nigel Godson, New York University School of Medicine: Figure 9.3

10. Edgar D. Rowton, Walter Reed Army Institute of Research: Figure 10.2
    Steven T. Brentano, University of Iowa: Figure 10.3
    Laurence Tetley and Keith Vickerman, University of Glasgow: Figure 10.4
    Klaus M. Esser, Walter Reed Army Institute of Research: Figure 10.5
    Don C. Wiley, Harvard University: Figure 10.9

12. Quesda/Burke, courtesy of Washington National Records Center: Figures 12.1 and 12.4
    U. S. Army: Figures 12.2, 12.3 and 12.5

INDEX

Page number in *italics* indicate illustrations.